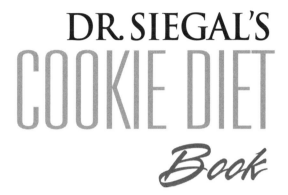

# DR. SIEGAL'S
# COOKIE DIET
## Book

# DR. SIEGAL'S
# COOKIE DIET
## *Book*

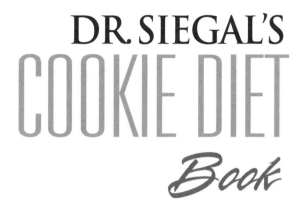

### HOW A DOCTOR
### AND HIS COOKIE
### HELPED 500,000 PEOPLE
### LOSE WEIGHT FAST

# SANFORD SIEGAL, D.O., M.D.

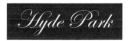

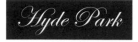

Published by Hyde Park Publishing Ltd., LLC
12254 SW 131st Avenue
Miami, FL 33186
888-870-0213 (U.S., toll-free)
001 202-664-1172 (Worldwide)
www.CookieDiet.com

Notice

This book is intended for entertainment and reference only, not as a medical manual. It is not intended to be used to diagnose or treat any medical condition or disease. You should consult your doctor before starting any weight-loss program or making any changes to your diet.

Jacket Photography: Oscar Borsten© 2008 SM Licensing Corp.
Book Design: Ghislain Viau
Book Jacket: Pablo Mejia
Book Coordination: Ellen Reid
Acknowledgements: Helen Durkin, Andrea Guerrieri, Pamela Howe, Peter Nguyen, Tanya Rivera, Lyndol Siegal, Matthew Siegal, Bruce Tracy, and hundreds of thousands of Dr. Siegal's Cookie Diet success stories

Publisher's Cataloging-in-Publication Data

Siegal, Sanford.

    Dr. Siegal's cookie diet book : how a doctor and his cookie helped
    500,000 people lose weight fast / Sanford Siegal ; foreword by
    Matthew Siegal. -- 1st. -- Miami, FL : Hyde Park Ltd., 2009.

        p. ; cm.

        ISBN: 978-0-9822728-3-1
        Includes bibliographical references and index.
        "The doctor's proven, three-step plan for safe, fast, and hunger-free
    weight loss."--Cover.

        1. Reducing diets. 2. Low-calorie diet. 3. Diet. 4. Health.
    I. Siegal, Matthew. II. Title. III. How a doctor and his cookie helped
    500,000 people lose weight fast.

RM222.2 .S54 2009                2009927481
613.25--dc22                   0908

10  9  8  7  6  5  4  3  2

*To Josie Raper, who is half her former size yet twice the person for sharing her story with the world and inspiring others to change their lives.*

# Contents

# Section Three

# Section Four

# Section Five

# Notices

This book makes reference to a weight-loss diet that is based on the consumption of 1,000 calories per day. That amount is only a suggestion to your doctor and you who, together, must decide what your daily caloric intake should be based on your medical history and examination. Only your doctor is qualified to determine whether a particular diet—or any diet—is right for you. Your doctor may raise or lower the suggested number of calories or advise you not to follow this diet. To ensure your success and health, consult your doctor before starting any diet and follow his advice.

## Proprietary Products

The Dr. Siegal's Cookie Diet weight-loss approach described in this book involves adhering to a reduced-calorie dietary regimen while controlling your hunger with Dr. Siegal's Cookie Diet brand cookies and shake mixes. These products are available online at CookieDiet.com and from select doctors, drug stores, and other retailers worldwide.

## For Patients of Siegal Medical Group

If you're a patient of Dr. Siegal's South Florida medical practice, Siegal Medical Group, this book will increase your understanding of

Dr. Siegal's Cookie Diet. However, this book is a book, not a doctor, and it does not give medical advice. At all times, you should carefully follow the instructions of your Siegal Medical Group physician.

## He or She

In this book, the pronoun "she" is used more frequently than the more common "he." That's because the majority of Dr. Siegal's Cookie Diet customers are women. If the English language, like some others, had a gender-neutral pronoun, the  author would gladly use it.

## Trademarks

To make this book more readable, the use of trademark symbols (™ and ®) to identify intellectual property has been avoided in most cases. Dr. Siegal's®, Dr. Siegal's Cookie Diet®, Hunger Wrecks Diets™, Cookie Doctor®, and the name and likeness of Dr. Sanford Siegal are trademarks of SM Licensing Corporation. All other trademarks are the property of their respective owners.

## Contacting Dr. Siegal's Direct Nutritionals, LLC (CookieDiet.com)

To order Dr. Siegal's Cookie Diet brand products, or for assistance using Dr. Siegal's Weight-Loss Calculators, visit CookieDiet.com or call 877-377-4342 (from North America) or 001 703-677-8068 (from elsewhere).

# Foreword

My father is Dr. Sanford Siegal, the famous "Cookie Doctor" whom we see on TV and read about in newspapers and magazines, and I'm Matthew Siegal, the CEO of the Dr. Siegal's Cookie Diet retail businesses. I wasn't always involved in the cookie business, of course. I was barely out of diapers when my father conceived the idea of a weight-loss system based on a hunger-satisfying cookie. But I was always aware of it. I grew up in Miami, where Siegal Medical Group, my father's medical practice, is based. Where I came from, just about everyone knew about the doctor whose cookies helped people lose weight. The first TV show to profile my father and his cookie was *Montage*, a local TV newsmagazine. That was in 1985, and I remember being very proud the day that everyone at school was talking about seeing my father on TV.

I went off to college with the idea of becoming a lawyer, but on the very first day my plans changed. I discovered the personal computer and was instantly smitten. During that same year, after buying a book about computer programming, I started my own software company. I remained enrolled in college for several more years but never took it seriously. I skipped a lot of classes. My software company was growing fast, and I was having a blast running it. School? A lawyer? Yeah, right.

After a few years, I dropped out of college, sold my first software company, and started a second one. Eleven years later, I sold my second company to my first one and stayed on as a senior executive. Two years later, in 2005, the company went public in a particularly successful initial public offering. By early 2008, the company that started in a college kid's apartment had a market capitalization of $700 million and was traded on NASDAQ. And that's when I quit my job there and launched the retail side of Dr. Siegal's Cookie Diet.

It's not that I was unhappy as a software company executive. On the contrary, for an entrepreneur with a genuine love of business, being on the management team of a publicly traded company was thrilling. But several factors combined to motivate me to go from making software that helps people grow their bottom lines to making cookies that help them reduce their bottoms (and other parts). Chief among these factors was that, for the first time in more than 30 years, my father's reputation as the creator of what was then commonly known as "the cookie diet" was under attack. Indeed, it seemed to me that his weight-loss system was in serious jeopardy of being hijacked by opportunistic entrepreneurs.

There were also other, more personal reasons for my sudden career change. For one, a number of years earlier, I had personally benefited from Dr. Siegal's Cookie Diet.

About 10 years ago, I was sitting in a restaurant in Tampa with my father who was there for a medical conference. I had flown down from my home in Maryland to join him for the weekend because, frankly, I was feeling terrible and needed the company. I was noticeably distraught and had been for some time. At one point during the meal, my father reached across the table, took my wrist, and began to check my pulse. About 15 seconds later he said, "Matt, you have the slowest pulse I've taken on anyone who wasn't dead." After a moment or two, he continued. "You're depressed for no apparent reason, and you're a good 40 pounds overweight. I suspect hypothyroidism."

It turned out that he was right. But we'll get to that in a moment.

Until my senior year of high school, I was a svelte kid and a happy one. But then I began to gain weight. At 5'8", I quickly went from about 140 pounds to 155 pounds. By my sophomore year of college, I was at least 30 pounds overweight, and a couple of years later, I was at 187 pounds, the heaviest I had ever been. At the same time that my weight went north, my spirits went south. I'd been a happy-go-lucky kid until around the twelfth grade; then my mood changed. I became less active and more reclusive.

You're probably thinking that my increasing weight had a negative effect on my mood and undoubtedly it did to some extent. Certainly, I was too depressed to care about my appearance and so I neglected it. But why did I allow myself to become overweight in the first place? Of my excess weight and my depression, which was cause and which was effect?

While being overweight contributed to my unhappiness, it wasn't the root cause. Nor was anything going on in my life to explain it. On the contrary, life was good. The software company I'd founded during my freshman year was doing very well. I felt that I was on my way to being the next Bill Gates and loved being in that position. Indeed, I would have been the happiest person alive were it not for the fact that on many days I wanted to be dead.

Now, let's return to that restaurant in Tampa. Somewhere between salad and dessert (my dessert, of course, not his; the Cookie Doctor doesn't eat dessert, at least not in public!), my father concluded, based on my very low pulse rate, my appearance, and my state of mind, that I had a sluggish metabolism. A short time later, he gave me a prescription for thyroid medication.

I returned to Maryland and continued to take my thyroid pills. I also took my father's advice to go on a diet. I don't think he specifically tied that advice to my mental state; he just felt that being 40 pounds overweight was a bad idea. To help me drop the weight, he started sending me boxes of the hunger-controlling cookies he'd been dispensing to his patients for many years.

Before long, I went from 187 pounds to 140 pounds and looked great.[1] I also felt great. Whereas just months earlier it had been a struggle to pull myself out of bed in the morning, I now leaped from bed (often before the alarm rang), eager to start a new day.

That was a decade ago, and I still usually wake up feeling that way.

There's one more reason I'm now involved with Dr. Siegal's Cookie Diet. About two years ago, the Fox News Channel sent a TV crew to Miami to do a segment about my father. For fun, I flew down to observe. The crew was in my father's clinic for hours, during which time many patients came and went. Toward the end of the shoot, the lights and camera were pointed at my father and the producer was asking him questions. I was standing near him, just out of view of the camera. Suddenly, from the other side of the office where the door to the waiting room stood open, a woman came running toward us with her arms open. Before I could react, she had pushed her way past the cameraman and literally (I swear, I'm not exaggerating) wrapped her arms around my father and, with tears coming down her cheeks, kept repeating, "Thank you, Dr. Siegal. Thank you." It turns out that the woman, who had been a patient for some time but had never met my father (he has other doctors who work with him), had been a yo-yo dieter all her life before finally losing the weight at Siegal Medical Group.

This Kodak moment made a real impression on me (and on everyone else in the room, for we were all a bit misty-eyed). I'd spent

---

[1] Most people thought I looked great. My mother literally gasped in horror the first time she saw me minus 40-some pounds. "Oh no! My baby's dying!" she cried. And a few weeks later, when I had hit my goal weight of 140 pounds, my brother, Jason, confronted me and said, "OK, enough is enough. This is an intervention." Fortunately, both of them quickly got over the shock of seeing me at a healthful weight.

my entire adult life selling really good software to companies that genuinely benefited from it. And while I had received a lot of compliments from clients over the years, I sure couldn't recall any of them having been moved to tears by my software.

While the woman was still hugging him and thanking him, my father looked at me over his shoulder and, seeming to be pleased with himself, said, "You know, there are worse ways to make a living."

Indeed.

Matthew Siegal, CEO
Dr. Siegal's Direct Nutritionals, LLC
McLean, VA
April 2009

# Introduction

It took me 15 years to write this book. I wrote a significant part of it in the early 1990s and then became distracted by other projects, including another book, *Is Your Thyroid Making You Fat?* (Warner Books, 2000). I added chapters here and there over the next decade or so but never quite managed to finish. My 2007 New Year's resolution was to wrap it up by that summer. But I was happily sidetracked for a good year by the launch of the retail side of Dr. Siegal's Cookie Diet. Finally, with all that out of the way, I buckled down in the summer of 2008 and began the last leg of my literary journey.

This book is divided into five sections. I hope you'll read all of them because, in my half century in practice, I've learned that the more informed my patients are, the more likely they are to succeed. I suspect that the same is true of diet book readers so, do yourself a favor, please read the whole book.

Sections 1 and 4 are the most important parts of the book if you intend to follow Dr. Siegal's Cookie Diet and wish to get the best results. They explain the basic concept of my weight-loss approach and provide instructions for following the diet.

Section 5 contains just one chapter, Chapter 23, and is intended for your doctor to read. Throughout the book I advise you to consult your doctor before starting any diet. If you bring him the book and he reads the chapter I wrote for him, your consultation with him may be more fruitful.

The bulk of the pages you hold in your hand are found in Sections 2 and 3 which, in my opinion, are the most interesting and entertaining parts of the book, and the most scholarly. As you read these sections, you'll discover that I devote a significant portion of the book to discussing a dietary regimen that I don't, in fact, advocate for my patients or for you. It's a diet consisting mainly of meat and fat. Yes, you read correctly. I talk a lot about a diet in which one eats liberal quantities of meat and fat as a means of losing weight, and yet I don't recommend such a diet for anyone.

In Sections 2 and 3, you'll learn that a sizable and diverse group of respected doctors, scientific researchers, anthropologists, and even a great Arctic explorer—some from decades or centuries past, others from modern times—have adhered to and extolled the virtues of such a diet.

Why, you may ask, do I discuss in great detail a diet that I don't endorse? The short answer is that, while I don't believe that "meat diets" are the correct answer to the question of what is the best diet for safe and effective weight loss, I discovered long ago that they provide valuable clues, clues that led me to create a hunger-controlling food more than 34 years ago.

If you don't know it already, Dr. Siegal's Cookie Diet, the weight-loss approach that I created in 1975, is based on a special cookie that I engineered to control my patients' hunger and help them stick to the low-calorie diet that I favor. The inspiration for my cookie was the considerable body of evidence—some anecdotal, some the result of formal studies—that diets comprising as much as 80 percent fatty meat have proven to be effective for weight reduction. Early in my career, I was skeptical of these diets because they ran counter to what I was taught in medical school. But as I read more and more on the subject, I eventually concluded that there were simply too many people, too many stories, to dismiss them.

Obviously, there was something about meat that was causing people to lose weight, although no one had identified it.

In the early 1960s, I became aware of a body of work that suggested that diets of meat and fat were useful in eliminating excess weight. Since that time, I've read countless papers, books, and newspaper articles on the subject of meat diets. I've spent innumerable hours poring over dusty volumes in medical libraries. I've even tracked down and interviewed the widows of some of the earlier advocates of these diets.

I can't say with certainty why eating meat has helped people lose weight, but I'm convinced it has. It's well established that certain food substances (such as proteins) do a better job of satisfying hunger than others (such as carbohydrates). I believe that certain components of meat are especially effective. Chief among these is fat. Maybe fat does such a good job of controlling hunger that people eat less when on a meat diet.

Fortunately, we don't need to eat lots of meat and fat to benefit from their hunger-satisfying properties. The mixture of proteins in my cookie does the job nicely without the high amount of calories, cholesterol, and fat found in meat. My cookie, although it looks, smells, and tastes like a cookie, is a lot like meat. It contains a variety of proteins derived from meat. In creating my protein formula, my goal was to engineer a food that contained the hunger-controlling components of meat without the possibly "bad" stuff that goes with it. It was my hope, and later my belief, that it was something in meat—not the entire slab of ribs—that satisfied hunger. I believe that the results enjoyed by those who have used my cookie over the years support my position.

Now you know why I devote so much of this book to meat and fat even though the actual "diet" part of this book has little to do with meat eating. I had to prove to you that I didn't pull the concept behind Dr. Siegal's Cookie Diet out of a hat. I based it on the experiences and research of many respected authorities. If you're going to ask people to take a leap of faith, to trust you when you tell them that they will lose weight by eating cookies all day, you have a responsibility to earn that trust, to demonstrate that you know what you're talking about.

By the way, I know why you bought this book, or are about to buy it. Don't believe me? Well, I'll tell you. I could give you a long explanation, one that's based on my 50 years of experience treating and observing the behavior of more than 500,000 overweight patients. But I won't do that to you. I don't have that much time, and neither do you. Instead, I'll condense the explanation into two words: cookie diet.

The name Dr. Siegal's Cookie Diet is both a blessing and a curse. Without its cute name you might never have heard of my weight-loss system. Yet there's no doubt that any approach that combines the words "cookie" and "diet" risks being branded a fad or gimmick. But fear not. I promise you, Dr. Siegal's Cookie Diet is a serious, proven system that has been used successfully by medical doctors for decades. With that kind of history behind it, if it's a fad, then it must be among the longest-running fads in history.

Given the media frenzy over Dr. Siegal's Cookie Diet, you may be familiar with the nickname that the media and the public bestowed upon me back in 1975: "The Cookie Doctor." I used to dislike that name but lately I've come to accept it. The reason I objected to that moniker in the past was that it suggests that Dr. Siegal's Cookie Diet, the thing for which I am best known, is the sum total of my contribution to the study and treatment of overweight problems. It isn't. Over the past 50 years, I've learned an awful lot about diagnosing and treating the problems of the overweight patient. I've shared my knowledge with the world in books I've written. These include one of the very first books to claim health benefits for diets high in fiber and low in refined sugar and flour (1975); the only diet book I know of devoted to the subject of controlling hunger without drugs (1985); and a controversial book about the devastating effects of hypothyroidism and the all-too-common failure of my fellow physicians to spot the condition in their overweight patients (2000).

At some point, however, I realized that no single name could adequately reflect the output of work from a 50-year (and counting!) medical career. Would I have preferred to be called the High Fiber Diet Pioneer? The Hypothyroidism Diagnosis and Treatment Contrarian? Alas, no. Those names are no more all-encompassing—and not nearly as memorable—as The Cookie Doctor.

Okay, so Dr. Siegal's Cookie Diet is going to be my legacy. At 80 years of age I'm now completely comfortable with that fact. While I hope that my books have contributed to a broader understanding of excess weight and how to reduce it, it is my cookie that has benefited the greatest number of people, and that will continue to do so after I'm gone. I'm proud to have helped so many people reach a more healthful weight and improve the quality of their lives.

The diet on which you are about to begin (with your doctor's approval) really works. I won't try to kid you, though. Under the best of circumstances, following a regimen that truly results in the loss of fat in a reasonable period of time is nobody's idea of fun. But if you follow my suggestions and, just as important, those of your doctor, you'll reach your goal as fast as possible, safely, and without hunger.

Here's to your health and success.

Sanford Siegal, D.O., M.D.
Miami, Florida
April 2009

# Section One

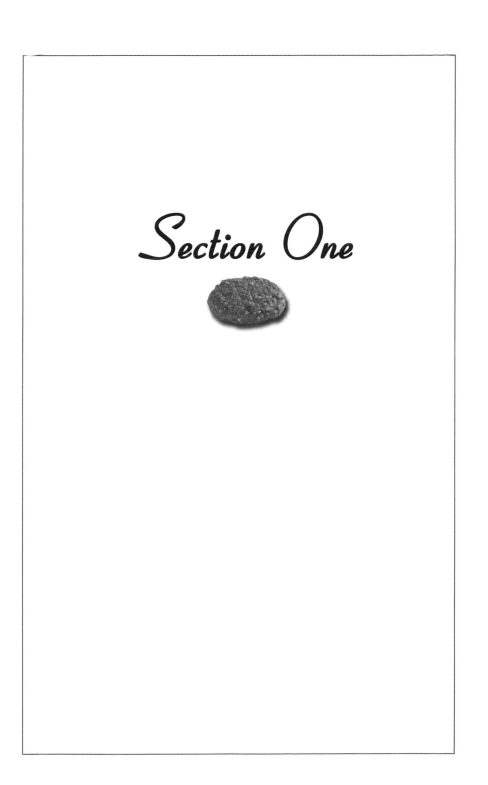

*Chapter 1*

# Lifestyle Changes

As the creator of a weight-loss system with a name as catchy as Dr. Siegal's Cookie Diet, I am always prepared for knee-jerk criticism or even summary dismissal by those who simply can't get beyond the name and learn the facts about my approach. Sometimes the criticism I hear is downright childish and based solely on the name. For example:

*"Eating cookies to lose weight? Sign me up and pass the Oreos!"*

*"Here we go again, another fad diet."*

Sometimes, however, the criticism is a bit more sophisticated if, ultimately, unfounded.

*"By advocating such a low-calorie regimen, Dr. Siegal's Cookie Diet will certainly make you lose weight but the results won't be permanent because it isn't a lifestyle change. Only a lifestyle change can keep the weight off permanently."*

Without a doubt, that argument—that Dr. Siegal's Cookie Diet doesn't promote a change of lifestyle that supports lifetime weight maintenance—is the most common made against my approach and others that result in fast weight loss due to a low-calorie dietary regimen. If you think *I'm* going to summarily dismiss *that* argument you're in for a surprise. Like the eighteenth- and nineteeth-century figures whose writings influenced my own research and led me to create my hunger-controlling cookie (more on that in later chapters), those who charge that my system does not promote permanent weight loss have reached an incorrect conclusion, yet the reasoning that led them to it has some merit. Specifically, their emphasis on lifestyle change as the key to permanent weight loss is absolutely correct. But in dismissing Dr. Siegal's Cookie Diet as a "fad diet," they fail to recognize two facts: (1) how we lose weight and how we maintain it are necessarily different, and (2) my diet (and nearly every other reduced-calorie diet) clearly requires one to make a lifestyle change.

To understand why these detractors reached wrong conclusions through partially correct reasoning, we must clarify what is meant by "lifestyle change." In my medical practice, we've treated more than 500,000 overweight patients during the past 50 years. All of these folks became overweight in exactly the same way: they ate too much. Some (especially the approximately 25 percent who had a metabolic problem) undoubtedly became overweight by eating just a little too much, perhaps very few calories a day more than was required to maintain their weight. But most ate way too much. I've had patients over the years who admitted to consuming 5,000, 8,000, and even 10,000 calories a day. I've seen many patients heavier than 300 pounds and a few heavier than 500. (If you've ever wondered why people who eat 10,000 calories a day never reach 2,000 pounds, see Chapter 12.)

Nobody starts out very overweight. Sure, some babies arrive bigger than others but nobody is born carrying around an extra 50 pounds. Furthermore, nobody puts on an extra 50 pounds overnight. They do it gradually by overeating for months or even years. They do it by living a particular *lifestyle*, one in which they eat more than is needed to maintain their weight. Let's be clear: the way we become overweight is by maintaining a lifestyle in which we eat more than we need and, in most cases, exercise less than we should.

To illustrate the kind of lifestyle that leads to a serious weight problem, let's imagine a fictional person, Bob, who is 5'10" and 275 pounds, a good 100 pounds overweight. What kind of lifestyle do you think Bob has led to reach his present weight? Would you be surprised if a typical day in Bob's life included a drive-thru bacon and egg croissant with hash browns for breakfast; a juicy steak, mashed potatoes, and all-you-can-eat salad bar at the steak-house where he entertains clients over lunch; a few cups of coffee with half-and-half throughout the day; half a pizza or his wife's wonderful meatloaf with mac and cheese for dinner; and a few scoops of ice cream in front of the tube before bed? Well, don't be surprised, because I've seen thousands of "Bobs" in my practice and I expect to see many more.

By the way, do you know what usually gets people like Bob to put down the burrito and go on a diet? All too often, it's the heart attack of a friend of a similar age and lifestyle. It's true. In my practice, women usually come to me because they want to look better. The men are afraid of dropping dead in their 50s like someone they knew.

So his friend has a heart attack, which scares Bob into action. He resolves to drop the spare tire and start hitting the gym again. To lose the weight, he decides to try that doctor's funny-sounding diet with the cookies that he keeps hearing about in the news. So he orders the cookies online or buys them from his own doctor or a local store. He opens the box and reads the instructions. During the day, with his doctor's blessing, he's to eat six 90 calorie cookies and absolutely nothing else except zero calorie beverages. At night, he's to eat a small dinner consisting of a few ounces of lean chicken, turkey, or fish and a cup of steamed green vegetables.

Keep in mind what Bob's menu has been for a very long time until this moment. We're talking about a guy who's used to eating 3,000 calories, 100 grams of fat, and 300 grams of sugar and starch every day. But starting today, he's going to nibble six good but not great-tasting cookies and nothing else all day. Each morning, he's going to drive past the drive-thru window without stopping. At lunch time, he'll satisfy his hunger with a cookie or two while his clients at the same table feast on prime sirloin. Mercifully, we'll allow him to continue drinking his several cups of coffee throughout the day except with one big change: he'll use no whitener, not even skim milk, let alone half-and-half. For dinner, Bob will enjoy an adequate but modest serving of lean poultry or fish, along with some non-starchy veggies. Instead of the ice cream he's used to having before bed, he'll have to settle for—well—nothing.

Do you get the point? Anyone who compares Bob's old regimen with the one he follows on Dr. Siegal's Cookie Diet and still argues that a lifestyle change has not occurred is probably being disingenuous and, perhaps, has an ulterior (and likely commercial) motive. Of course it's a lifestyle change, a dramatic one. Or, are the naysayers hung up on the point that they will certainly make after reading the preceding paragraph or two: that even if it is a lifestyle change, it isn't a permanent one. Nobody can eat such a restrictive and low-calorie diet forever, they'll insist.

They're right, of course, but who told them it was *permanent?* They didn't hear it from me. The six-cookie, 1,000 calorie diet that I advocate for the average overweight person is a weight-*loss*, not a weight-*maintenance*, diet. It is intended to take you from an overweight state to a normal one as quickly as possible, safely, and without unreasonable hunger. Once the weight is off, I shift gears and propose a permanent lifestyle change that includes exercise and sensible eating for lifetime weight maintenance. The two phases involved are, of course, different. A diet that takes off weight is certainly different from a diet that maintains weight.

At the beginning of this chapter I said that losing weight and maintaining weight require different approaches. To be sure, each requires a lifestyle change, but not quite the same one. One change is temporary; the other permanent. In Chapter 22, we'll discuss lifelong weight maintenance.

There's another point I must make about the half-baked views that so many critics espouse about fast weight loss and its bearing on long-term weight maintenance. First, I'll make a confession: not every person who reaches a normal weight on Dr. Siegal's Cookie Diet keeps it off. Many, in fact, gain it back. Based on a half century of experience and observation, I believe that my approach is more successful than any in effecting long-term results, yet it's far from perfect. Human nature is human nature and I haven't found a way to change it. If people go back to the bad habits—the lifestyle—that made them overweight, nothing that Dr. Siegal or anyone else says, writes, or does will keep them from regaining the weight.

Let's return for a moment to our fictional character, Bob. If the major change of lifestyle that Bob made in faithfully adhering to Dr. Siegal's Cookie Diet resulted in his dropping his extra 100 pounds in, say, 10 months, wouldn't a reasonable person give credit to my system for facilitating his achievement? Of course! They'd slap me on the back and congratulate me on a job well done. And wouldn't they continue to applaud for as long as Bob kept the weight off? I think so.

But what would they say if, perhaps a year or two down the road, Bob's weight were to start to creep back up? Would they attribute his expanding waistline to Bob's actions or would they point the finger at the method (in this case, a low-calorie diet facilitated by a hunger-controlling cookie) that Bob used to shed his 100 pounds and achieve a normal weight? I think you'll agree that the culprit is Bob and not the weight-loss program that he followed successfully some time ago. If you do agree, you're probably in the minority. All you have to do is watch the many TV shows I've been on with nutritionists and other "experts" (there are links to these shows on the *In The News* section of CookieDiet.com) to see that many people irrationally blame Bob's recidivism on the method that took him to a normal weight rather than the actions that he took months or years later.

To illustrate the absurdity of this reasoning, imagine that you are an avid racquetball player who one day slipped during a game and broke your arm. You went to an orthopedist who set your fracture and put you in a cast for three weeks. A month after the cast came off you returned to the court, good as new. Then, a year later, you again slipped during a game and, alas, broke your arm. Would you go back to the same doctor who fixed you up last time? Or, would you blame your broken appendage on that doctor? Would you argue that the method that successfully healed your last broken arm was flawed because it did not permanently protect your arm from future racquetball mishaps?

It's a rhetorical question if ever there was one.

One doesn't fault the doctor or method that fixed a broken arm if one later breaks the arm again. Likewise, we shouldn't blame the doctor, dietician, fitness guru, or friend whose approach caused our weight to come off if we return to our old ways and gain it back.

I'm sure you've heard that if you lose it fast you gain it back just as fast. What nonsense! There is no correlation between how fast we lose weight and whether or not we keep it off. Once the weight comes off, your body doesn't remember how it was accomplished. It doesn't know whether it was Dr. Siegal's Cookie Diet or Weight Watchers or the Miracle Suppository Diet that was responsible. No matter how the weight was lost, the weight loser faces the very same very real task: to maintain it. Losing weight and maintaining weight—each requires a lifestyle change; the first is temporary, the other is permanent. Dr. Siegal's Cookie Diet helps you accomplish both.

## Chapter 2

# 500,000 Anecdotes

On June 20, 2008, the national Fox TV program *The Morning Show with Mike & Juliet* did a live segment about Dr. Siegal's Cookie Diet. I've done a lot of TV show appearances and this was among the best. The producer did a thorough research job. You can tell that from the accuracy of the two-minute video that aired at the beginning of the piece.

The segment featured four guests besides me. Seated to my left was a young woman from Arizona named Josie who in a short time had lost more than 100 pounds—nearly half her body weight—by following my diet under her doctor's supervision. Beside her was her mother, Yvonne, who admitted that she thought her daughter was "insane" when she first announced she'd be eating cookies while dieting. But within a month, Yvonne explained, she saw how fast the weight was falling off of Josie, and she joined her on the diet. By the time they appeared on the Fox show several months later, Yvonne had lost about 50 pounds.

There were two other guests on the show. To my right was a doctor, and next to him, a young nutritionist. What was their role?

They were there to disagree with me, regardless of what I said. Huh? I'll explain.

I've never taken a journalism class, but I'm pretty sure that on the first day of Journalism 101 they teach you that, to make a story appear to be balanced and fair, you have to find an "expert" to offer a view that is contrary to whatever view the main subject of the interview espouses. In almost every media interview I've ever done (and I've done more than 100 of them), the producer or editor has brought in a so-called expert to give the contrarian point of view. Usually they invite a nutritionist who appears to be fresh out of school. On rare occasions they find a doctor, often one who has never treated a patient for excess weight.

For my *Mike & Juliet* appearance, they seemed to have both.

The doctor who sat next to me was not an obesity specialist. Rather, as near as I could determine, his claim to fame was a book he'd written about bird flu. But that didn't stop him from attacking (loudly!) my diet and me. He began by saying that he hopes that he'll "have the good sense to be retired before I'm [Dr. Siegal's] age." (I share that hope.) He then went on to say that the 800 calorie diet that I have used in my practice for 34 years is extremely dangerous and will cause such terrifying side effects as bleeding, muscle loss, heart disease, and mental impairment. Had the segment been longer, he might have included bubonic plague, dropsy, pleurisy, dengue fever, and mange. "The body needs fuel! The body needs fuel!" he repeatedly screamed at me. (By the way, I resisted the temptation to offer the bird flu doctor a cookie and point out that *his* body, in fact, clearly needed *less* fuel.)

At one point during his tirade, I asked him if he had ever encountered a single person who had any problem with Dr. Siegal's Cookie Diet. He admitted that he hadn't but then added that he had "heard of people who have had problems." He didn't give any details, though, and immediately changed the subject.

Toward the end of the segment, I turned to Josie and asked if she had experienced bleeding, muscle loss, or heart disease. She said no and added that her doctor routinely monitored her and found her to be in excellent health. The other doctor, hoping to get in the last word, yelled at me, "But that's anecdotal evidence! It's anecdotal!" I replied, "Right, 500,000 anecdotes." Thus ended the segment.

Within 24 hours of the first airing of that segment (it was included in a "Best of Mike & Juliet" show a couple of months later), more than 6,000 viewers had registered on CookieDiet.com. Dozens of people had also e-mailed or called us to say that they were upset at how the other doctor had "beaten up" on poor Dr. Siegal. I was genuinely touched by the outpouring of support. (If you were one of the people who contacted us, thank you.)

Obnoxious as he was, the good doctor was right about one thing: my "evidence," indeed my entire approach to weight loss and to the formula in the cookies, is based on anecdotal evidence, not ivory tower research. Unlike data, which is the result of highly structured studies performed (one hopes) under tightly controlled conditions, anecdotal evidence is based simply on the observations of the one who compiles it.

But don't knock anecdotal evidence. Many important medical advances have resulted from it. Furthermore, consider the value of hands-on experience as you ponder this rhetorical question: If you needed to have your appendix removed or your clogged artery cleared, would you prefer that the surgery be performed by an ivory tower scholar who had never actually operated on anyone or an experienced surgeon, one who had performed thousands of operations similar to yours but perhaps had never authored a research paper?

Of course, I'm not saying that I pulled all of my beliefs out of a hat. There is certain data that is universally accepted and upon which I rely. For example, it is generally believed that approximately

3,500 excess calories produce a pound of fat. (Actually, I cautiously rely on that fact; I have a few reservations. See Chapter 12.) Furthermore, a good part of this book is devoted to the observations of earlier physicians, scientists, and laypeople whose views have influenced my own.

We humans love data, especially numbers. The more complex and hard to understand, the better. Charts, graphs, footnotes . . . we love them too. Data makes us feel safe. It legitimizes our beliefs. It frees us from the burden and responsibility of using common sense and places on someone else the responsibility for our decisions.

You may think that I am dismissing the value and validity of data. I'm not. I'm a physician, and certainly data is associated with every aspect of medicine. I also have a strong background in chemistry, and I went to engineering school too. I appreciate data.

By now you must be asking me, "So why haven't you bothered to support your views by conducting studies?" There are two reasons.

First, I can't afford to. No practicing physician can. Medical studies cost millions of dollars and are, therefore, done by large organizations, usually major universities. They're funded by industry, government, and charitable organizations. Few individuals or even single companies have the resources to fund a legitimate study. Certainly no private practice physician, no matter how successful, has such resources.

But there's another reason. What would I study? What hypothesis would I try to prove? I make exactly one claim for Dr. Siegal's Cookie Diet: My cookies control your hunger and help you stick to your diet.

The claim is, indeed, based on anecdotal evidence. How many anecdotes? There are about a half million. That's how many patients I've treated with Dr. Siegal's Cookie Diet during the past 34 years. And by the way, not one of them has had any serious problems with it. There's another important thing you should know about medical research data. At the risk of bursting your bubble, I must tell you that a lot of data that is presented as fact is simply wrong. Researchers do make mistakes. More important, however, data (especially medical data) is very often manipulated and distorted to support the interests of those who funded the research that produced it. There is no better example of this than the volumes of data produced by the tobacco industry over decades. Oh, have you forgotten? Smoking used to be good for you.

Getting back to anecdotal evidence, it's what your family doctor relies on when he sees the results of a particular procedure he follows in treating patients of a particular type or with a specific ailment. If he has adopted a method to help his patients, even though it differs from the "conventional" wisdom, and it produces positive results, he is basing his choice of treatment on anecdotal evidence. He invariably knows much more about his patient than the scientist who does research studies along the strict lines imposed by, say, a university-based project. The interaction with the subject in these formal studies is often cold and impersonal. Perhaps this approach is mandated in the interest of objectivity. One does not want his personal relationship with the subject to influence his observations or judgment.

Yet, when your family doctor helps you with a problem using his own seat-of-the-pants method and the result is good, how can we disparage it? Furthermore, if it seems to him that the same method has worked repeatedly on others with equally good results, does he not have a right, or even a duty, to continue to use that method?

I suspect that we have too much blind respect for reports that come from "experts" or "authorities" or prestigious institutions. Physicians who are overburdened with work, who don't have time to question the edicts that come down from the ivory towers, tend to accept anything that appears in print if the publication has known credentials.

I'm immediately reminded of a study that I read a few days ago in a very prestigious medical journal, *The New England Journal of Medicine.* Doctors with the highest credentials from the most respected institutions, including Harvard University, were associated with it. The idea was to determine whether one type of diet is better than another type. A large number of subjects was studied over a period of two years. They had been divided into four groups and the members of each group were instructed to eat a specific diet composed of certain amounts of protein, carbohydrate, and fat. The proportion of each of these nutrients was different for each of the four groups, and the total calories were adjusted so that they were equivalent for all of the subjects.

The subjects were not segregated or housed or monitored. There were no spies to verify their adherence. Therefore, presumably, the study's conclusions depended on the subjects' accurate and faithful adherence to the instructions given with respect to daily caloric intake and the distribution of those calories among protein, fat, and carbohydrates. In other words, the study relied on the honor system.

Researchers reported on the results six months into the experiment. The average weight loss overall was similar for the four groups. This led to the conclusion that the mixture of nutrients was not important to the result. Only the total calories counted.

The experiment was designed so that each subject would have a calorie deficit of 750 calories a day. Anyone professionally involved in weight loss (including I) knows that the 6 month weight loss in this case should have been about 38 pounds for each subject. As it turned out, the average weight loss was only 13 pounds. The report commented on that by saying that the amount of weight lost by all the subjects corresponded to an average intake of 500 calories a day more than each subject was instructed to eat. Clearly, the subjects did not follow the instructions they were given. Let's not get into honesty or motives or human frailties. The fact is that 800 people as a group did not do what the experiment required and yet the study was published, and its questionable conclusions presented as valid.

As far as I'm concerned, this was the most important finding—the subjects did not follow the prescribed diet. I would have ended the experiment right there, with the explanation that studies of eating behavior that rely on the honesty of the subjects are perhaps unreliable.

Instead, the study went on to conclude that, although the entire population of the four groups lost some weight, there was no difference in weight loss between groups based on the particular diet they had eaten. How did the researchers know what particular diet was eaten by each individual? If the subjects didn't or couldn't follow the instructions as to the number of calories they were supposed to eat, how could anyone believe that they meticulously followed the instructions as to measuring the amounts of protein, carbohydrate, and fat that they were instructed to eat?

Perhaps I'm being facetious, but should not a polygraph have been a part of the equipment used?

This is not an isolated criticism of a particular study. I have read many studies that had questionable conclusions or flawed techniques.

The results of the above study were reported throughout the media. The message: only calories count and it doesn't matter how you distribute them among various foods. That was already a universal belief. This study was meant to either substantiate or discredit that. It did neither.

I think the study offered more proof that investigations of human behavior that rely on the accurate reporting of the participants are simply unreliable. I think this is even more true when investigating people's eating habits. My patients love to tell me what they think I want to hear.

In my own case, after digesting a multitude of anecdotes, I believe that high protein diets in general are more effective for weight loss because they result in less hunger and therefore less intake of calories. The above study did nothing to change my opinion.

Anecdotes are little stories. Each of my patients supplies me with one of these stories. It has been said repeatedly that medicine is more an art than a science. Part of that art is to be able separate the truth in those stories from the untruths. You can't do that when there are only a handful of anecdotes. But by the time that hundreds of thousands of these anecdotes seem to confirm one another, you cannot help but believe that the information is potentially more valuable than that coming from flawed ivory tower research.

You'll learn much more about conventional medical studies in chapters to come.

One thing that everyone seems to agree on and that has been confirmed by countless studies is that being overweight is unhealthful and contributes to a host of serious medical problems. The world is filled with real people who have suffered real harm as a result of being overweight. The world is also filled with real people who used to be overweight and aren't anymore as a result of Dr. Siegal's Cookie Diet. Of course, that's anecdotal.

## Chapter 3

# Barbarians at the Oven Door

I believe in free enterprise, at least in principle, and no one ever said that an idea had to be original to make somebody a lot of money. But when it comes to Dr. Siegal's Cookie Diet and the growing number of "copycat" products it has spawned, I'm less enthusiastic. It's not that I mind competition, *per se*. It fuels innovation (well, sometimes); I can think of many good ideas that were made better by an enterprising entrepreneur.

Dr. Siegal's Cookie Diet isn't one of those ideas.

I've included this chapter (which I adapted from an entry I posted on my CookieDiet.com blog in April 2008) to help people distinguish between the original cookie-based diet that has received so much publicity and acceptance over the past three decades and those that have arrived very late to the party.

From 1975 to 2002, Dr. Siegal's Cookie Diet existed without significant copiers. Yes, over the years, there actually were a few half-hearted attempts to capitalize on my idea. For example, in the early 1980s, there was a doctor to whom I'd been supplying my cookies for use in his own practice. He bought a lot of cookies; then suddenly the weekly orders stopped coming. I soon learned that the budding entrepreneur in him had awakened and decided that he could make more money by stealing my idea than buying my cookies. Fortunately for me he was wrong. Nobody wanted his cookies because that's all they were—garden-variety cookies. In addition to underestimating the complexity of food manufacturing, he forgot one important thing. The reason Dr. Siegal's Cookie Diet works is that the cookies satisfy hunger without the usual calories that are found in common snacks. The particular mixture of proteins (with the particular distribution of amino acids) incorporated and the method of combining the ingredients are a secret known only to my wife and me at this time. Many are surprised to hear that we, in solitude, with our own hands, combine some of the ingredients that go into every cookie, thus preserving the secrecy and the uniqueness of my product.

Of course, whenever a product is successful, there will be imitators. It took 30 years for them to start arriving on the scene, but today there are at least three companies that recently started to offer products or services that use the words *cookie diet* in their marketing.

## Six Cookies, One Meal a Day, and 800 Calories

The essence of my system as used in my practice is quite simple. First, my patient undergoes a typical medical history and examination, including an EKG and various laboratory tests. She (most of my patients are women) then begins an 800-calorie-a-day diet that includes six of my cookies (more on those in a moment).[1] During

---

[1] In my own practice, my patients follow an 800 calorie diet. For those who are not my patients, I advocate a 1,000 calorie diet, and this book is based on 1,000 calories (or more).

her first month on my diet, my patient carefully tracks her weight loss. At the end of the first 28 days, I use the data she has gathered and a test that I developed to help me assess whether she has a sluggish metabolism caused by a condition called hypothyroidism. I estimate that about one quarter of the patients who come to me have this condition but don't know it, though many suspect that something is wrong with them. It's difficult to lose weight if you have hypothyroidism, and yet it is easily corrected with medication. If you suspect that you have an underactive thyroid even though conventional lab tests and your own doctor say otherwise, see Chapter 13 or, for even more information, read my book, *Is Your Thyroid Making You Fat?* (Warner Books, 2000).

## Enter Smart for Life Weight Management Centers

In late 2001 I was contacted by a charismatic Canadian doctor who requested and received my permission to open weight-loss clinics called Siegal Weight Management (later renamed Siegal Smart for Life Weight Management Centers) that used my six-cookies-a-day weight-loss system and hunger-controlling foods. Based on his initial success, he came back to me and obtained the right, as my franchisee, to sell sub-franchises. Within a few years, there were dozens of Siegal Smart for Life centers in such metropolitan areas as Philadelphia, Boston, Los Angeles, Boca Raton, Tampa Bay, and Quebec.

An important part of my agreement with him was that his centers could not use any foods for weight loss other than mine. My system had been working very well for the last 27 years and I did not want its reputation to be tarnished with inferior products.

In August 2006, despite our agreement and the fact that Siegal Smart for Life was growing rapidly, I received a letter from him announcing the immediate end to our agreement. Suddenly, Siegal

Smart for Life was just Smart for Life and was offering its own brand of cookies, shakes, and soups. Thankfully, I never had shared my secret formula with that doctor, and it has, therefore, never been found in his products.

The story doesn't end there. It made the news, and if you're interested in the fascinating conclusion, I'll direct you to two excellent articles on the subject. The first was published in the April 17, 2008, issue of the Broward/Palm Beach edition of *New Times*. The lengthy article provides a remarkably detailed account of my entire relationship with that franchisor from the beginning up until the recent time (April 2008). The second article appeared in the November 17, 2008, issue of *Forbes* magazine. Links to both articles are posted under *In the News* on CookieDiet.com.

In September 2008, I learned from the Web site of the *South Florida Business Journal* that my former franchisee had filed for Chapter 11 bankruptcy protection.

## Hollywood Cookie Diet

As I recall, it was sometime in June 2006 that a self-proclaimed "diet guru" named Jamie Kabler began selling a box of cookies under the name Hollywood Cookie Diet. You may have heard of Kabler. He's the same fellow who previously brought you the Hollywood 48-Hour Miracle Diet (and later, perhaps for those in a hurry, the 24-Hour version). These earlier products are blends of fruit juices that have used "Lose Up to Five Pounds in 24 Hours" as a slogan. Now I'm just a practicing physician, not an ordained diet guru, but it seems to me that any juice that produces five pounds of weight loss in 24 hours is flushing away a lot of material of which body fat is not a significant component.

As for his so-called Hollywood Cookie Diet, I have to commend Kabler for not making false claims for it, at least as of this writing. In fact, except for occasional uses of words such as *miracle* and *magic,* I wasn't able to find any claims at all on his Web site. There's no specific information about how the cookies aid in weight loss. The product's marketing slogan is "The First Delicious Way to Lose Weight!"

If you believe that true weight loss can be achieved through magic, miracles, and the consumption of delicious foods, then I believe your prospect for success is the only thing that will ever be slim.

## And This Just in from Japan

Very recently a product called Soypal Cookie Diet popped up online. I don't know anything about it. However, I will infer from its name that it may contain soy protein. If that's the case, then beware of this. Based on my experience with my own patients, I estimate that low thyroid function is a contributing factor in the excess weight of about one in four overweight people. Why is that relevant? Because recent published studies have linked low thyroid hormone levels to the consumption of soy protein. For that reason, I have intentionally left soy protein out of all Dr. Siegal's Cookie Diet products.[2] Furthermore, in my own practice, we discourage patients from consuming soy protein.

## Cookies Don't Make People Lose Weight

Losing weight is nobody's idea of fun even under the best of circumstances. It takes discipline and determination to achieve your goal. I've used Dr. Siegal's Cookie Diet to help more than a half million people lose weight. The weight loss that those people experienced was not the result of eating cookies. It was the result

---

[2] On the Dr. Siegal's Cookie Diet product packaging you'll notice that I use soybean oil. There is no contradiction. According to the USDA National Nutrient Database for Standard Reference, soybean oil does not contain soy protein.

of adhering to a reduced-calorie diet that was made possible with the use of a particular cookie—my cookie.

## Conclusion

Free enterprise is alive and well in America. I expect more ersatz "cookie diets" to appear. I'll leave it to the consumers and to the patients to decide whether to trust the knockoffs or the real McCoy (or the real Siegal).

*Chapter 4*

# How to Keep a Secret

I'm frequently asked how my cookie can be made with a secret formula when, like all packaged foods, the ingredients are clearly listed on the label.

One answer I could give you would have to do with pointing out the secrecy of the Coca-Cola recipe. Every bottle or can of Coca-Cola lists the ingredients on the label, yet we all know that no one has ever been able to exactly duplicate Coca-Cola. We must assume that a lot of very smart people have tried and failed.

Here's a better way to explain it. I'm not going to tell you my secrets. Instead, to help you understand how it's possible to keep a formula a secret, I'm going to create a totally bogus scenario to make my point.

Let's rename you, my dear reader, Esmeralda. You, Esmeralda, are famous among your family and friends for the wonderful black pepper salad dressing you make. You keep its recipe a secret, but you generously give bottles of it to your family and friends on special occasions. They love it. No one knows your secret recipe, and you won't divulge it.

One day, your uncle says, "Why don't you bottle it and sell it to the grocery store down the street?" With that suggestion, "Esmeralda's Black Pepper Salad Dressing" is born.

You learn the rules about how to label a product for sale in stores. You've read that you must list the ingredients on the label. The rules say that they "shall be listed by common or usual name in descending order of predominance by weight." That's exactly what you're going to do. And yet you'll still be able to keep your secret.

Now let's pretend that I just happen to be the only other one who knows your secret recipe. Sorry, Esmeralda, but I'm now going to tell the world *your* secret formula, right now. Here's how you make your incomparable salad dressing.

You start with a half pound of black peppercorns. You know what those are. They're usually labeled "Whole Black Pepper." It's the stuff that's in those giant pepper mills in restaurants that only waiters use and won't let you get your hands on. (Obviously they don't trust you with it.)

You have an electric coffee grinder, and you use it not for coffee, but to finely grind your half pound of peppercorns. You dump the very fine black powder that you've made into a four-quart stainless-steel pot. To this you add one quart of your favorite olive oil. You cover it tightly and then place the pot on the front left burner of your electric stove and set the knob to low. You leave it cooking there for exactly two hours and 45 minutes. At that temperature it gets very hot, but it doesn't quite boil.

At the end of that time, you open the pot and pour in two quarts of vinegar. You mix the contents thoroughly. The stuff in the pot looks like a black mess. You heat it only for another five minutes. You then pour it through one of those paper coffee filters and collect the oily liquid that drips out very slowly into another clean, four-quart stainless-steel pot. That filtered liquid looks just like your famous salad dressing always looks. It's sort of yellowish and has a delightful odor. All that black goo that's left in the coffee filter is thrown in the garbage.

You now heat your dressing on medium and carefully time it while it boils. At five minutes, you remove it from the stove and cautiously pour this really hot stuff into the 10 clean bottles that you've had waiting. You immediately screw on the lids. It's done.

(At this point I must again emphasize that this entire recipe as well as the story is bogus. I just made it up. I doubt that this stuff would taste good or that it's even feasible to follow these instructions. For God's sake, don't actually try to make it! It will probably taste lousy. This is a phony example invented only to illustrate my point about keeping a formula a secret.)

Next you make some ugly labels on your home computer. As amateurish as they are, you've done your homework and they have all the proper information that the law requires.

One section of the label is most important. We see this section on thousands of products in the supermarket. It reads, "Ingredients."

Your ingredients section is very simple: vinegar, olive oil, black pepper. That's all. There's nothing about grinding and heating and boiling and filtering. Just three ingredients are all that went into Esmeralda's Black Pepper Salad Dressing. In the bottle, you can't see even a trace of the black pepper. The label is perfectly legal. For people to exactly duplicate your salad dressing, they'd have to make a lot of good guesses.

Now suppose some enterprising neighbor lady, Gwendolyn, decides to "knock off" Esmeralda's Black Pepper Salad Dressing. (Believe me it will happen; I have to contend with more than one "Gwendolyn.") After all, Gwendolyn knows the three ingredients; they're on the label. What she doesn't know is the process. She doesn't know about the grinding, the two-stage heating, and the filtering. So she simply mixes the three ingredients and pours it cold into bottles. She then lists the same three ingredients on the copy she's made of Esmeralda's label. The only thing she changes on the label is the name of the product.

We now have "Gwendolyn's Black Pepper Salad Dressing," a foul, black, gritty, gooey mess that no one can pour out of the bottle. If a few gullible souls buy a bottle, they'll never buy another.

Esmeralda, you've kept your secret.

The government obviously doesn't want us to give away our trade secrets. They simply want to protect the public. They believe the public has a right to know what goes into the things they eat. Esmeralda and I both follow the rules. Strangely enough, Gwendolyn also followed the rules.

God knows people have tried to pry out of me the information about my cookie. So far my wife, I, and a safe deposit box are the only ones who know it. Were I to have divulged it years ago, everyone would be brewing up a variation of it in their garages, making outlandish claims for what it could do, and soiling the reputation of my special product.

That's why it's still a secret.

Nonetheless, there are poor imitations of Dr. Siegal's cookie out there. But those copycats didn't even bother to try to copy the ingredients or even guess at the process. They weren't even as resourceful as Gwendolyn. They simply made ordinary cookies.

That's life!

*Chapter 5*

# Six Incorrect Things People Will Say about This Book

I know of no field of medicine that is as rife with nonsensical advice as that of nutrition. As I noted in Chapter 2, when I appear on a television news show, the producer usually invites a so-called expert to refute what I say, whatever it may be. On rare occasions the other guest is a physician, but in most cases she's a nutritionist (whatever that is) or a registered dietician, someone whose views are based not on her experience treating hundreds of thousands of patients, but rather on what she has read in textbooks. Still, these counter points of view add an illusion of objectivity to these shows and will always be a part of them.

Since I expect to devote a significant amount of time to doing media interviews to publicize this book, you might see me doing battle with such types on your favorite talk show or the local news. In this chapter I thought it would be useful to tell you what you can expect to hear from these detractors and to explain why it is, as the British say, *piffle*.

## 1,000 Calories Is Not Enough

Right! Of course it's not "enough," that's why you lose weight. There's no question about it: on 1,000 calories a day, everyone loses weight. When it comes to caloric intake, "enough" means enough to maintain your weight, and that's not what we're looking for in a weight-reduction diet.

## Losing Weight Fast Is Dangerous

Says who? And how long, dear expert, will it take for those ill effects to appear? It's been 34 years since I started the first of more than 500,000 patients on an 800 calorie diet, and I'm still waiting for the first sign of trouble. The 1,000 (or more) calorie diet that I advocate in this book takes off about 10 pounds per month and is safe.

## Dr. Siegal's Cookie Diet Doesn't Offer Enough Food Variety

This common allegation (which is never accompanied by an explanation as to its meaning) has always puzzled me. Enough variety for what? I remember one nutritionist saying that a diet where one eats cookies all day "sets people up for binge eating" or some such nonsense. That's rubbish. If anything, having a limited menu of good-tasting but not delicious foods discourages such aberrant behavior. It's no accident that the cookies I make for hunger control taste good but not great. If I were to make them taste too good, people would be more likely to eat more of them than necessary to control hunger. Having a seemingly endless array of delicious foods at our fingertips is what got 65 percent of us in the predicament we're in.

## If You Lose Weight Too Quickly, You're More Likely to Gain It Back

If you follow the news about diet and nutrition, this statement is among the most common you hear, and it's the most absurd. Your body does not know or remember how it lost weight or how fast. Whether you lose weight at a rate of ten pounds a month or ten pounds a year, the rate of loss is not a determining factor for whether you'll gain it back. What influences that is the eating and the exercise you do after you've lost the weight. To be more precise, the only factor in weight loss and weight gain is your net calories, the number of calories you take in from food less the number you burn up. If you return to the same bad habits that made you overweight in the first place, then you certainly will gain back the weight regardless of how quickly or slowly you lost it.

## Dr. Siegal's Cookie Diet Is a Fad Diet

All I can say is, "500,000 people, 34 years." If Dr. Siegal's Cookie Diet is a fad, someone should notify the *Guinness Book of World Records* because it's probably the longest-running fad in history.

## Dr. Siegal's Cookie Diet Isn't a Lifestyle Change

It most certainly is a lifestyle change, and a dramatic one at that. The lifestyle that leads to significant excess weight is in sharp contrast to the low-calorie, six-cookies-a-day-plus-dinner regimen required by Dr. Siegal's Cookie Diet. However, the lifestyle change that I advocate for weight *loss* is not the same as the one for weight *maintenance*. The former is a temporary, the latter, a permanent, lifestyle change. In this book, I explain in detail how Dr. Siegal's Cookie Diet results in both kinds of changes.

# Section Two

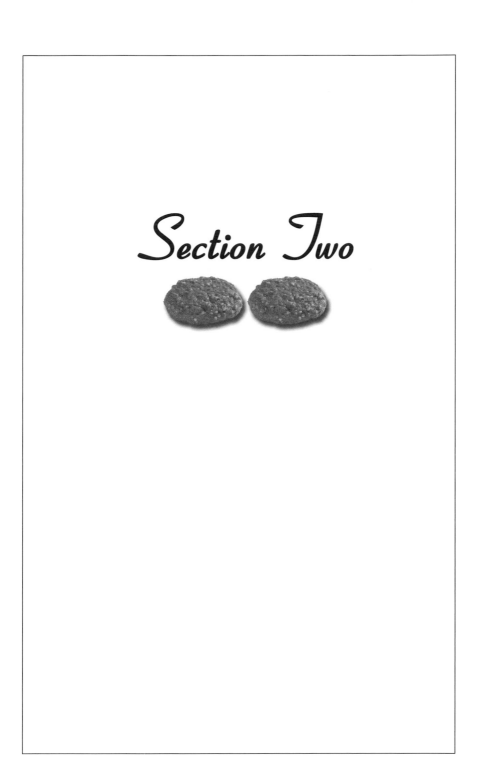

# Chapter 6
# Fat and the Human Race

You probably can't find a diet book that doesn't use the word *fat* many, many times. In our daily lives, we use the word repeatedly but with a variety of different meanings.

If your doctor were to tell you to stay away from fat, he would mean that you shouldn't eat foods fried in oil and to avoid butter, cheese, eggs, and most salad dressings, along with a lot of other "fat" things. But like many words, *fat* has acquired multiple definitions in our language. Many of the definitions assign a meaning that suggests excess. A fat book is a thick one. "Fathead" perhaps indicates an excess of stupidity. We say, "She's too fat," or, "I don't like to eat fat," or we may even express doubt by saying, "Fat chance." "Fatso" does not generally denote approval. A big corporation may try to "trim the fat" while the Bible speaks of "the fat of the land."

I've known for a long time that my patients get confused by the multiple meanings ascribed to certain words. I recall the frequent confusion over other common words such as *nerve* or *nervous*. My receptionist's opinion that Mrs. X has a lot of nerve has little to do with the nerve damage Mrs. X suffered in an auto accident. When the patient is told that the severe pain in his face is caused by a disorder of one of his cranial nerves, he may reply, "Yes, I've always been nervous," clearly demonstrating that he and the doctor are on different wavelengths. *Fat* is one of those confusing words.

Let's clear the air by looking into just what fat is and what is meant when the word is used in different ways. We will also have to look at other words that are quite naturally associated with it. In reading on the subject of fat, you frequently encounter such words as *suet, tallow, lard, oil, grease, shortening,* and even some that are less familiar such as *adipose.*

Let's get rid of the last one first. *Adipose* is simply medical jargon for the adjective, *fat.* If your doctor impresses you with the word "adipose," he is just talking about that loose layer of stuff around your middle or elsewhere that bobbles when you walk.

The fat on the bodies of cattle and hogs is much like the fat on your own body. It might more properly be called *fatty tissue* since it is one of the components, or "tissues," of animal bodies. You are certainly familiar with its appearance. There is plenty of it in the meat case of the supermarket. It's the off-white layer that surrounds a roast or a leg of lamb, it streaks your morning bacon, and is the many little white flecks in that raw steak. When cooked, its appearance changes somewhat. It gets shinier, more liquid, darker, less opaque, and certainly a lot softer than when it first came out of the refrigerator. Its normal state in the human body is really quite soft and mushy as opposed to the very firm feel of refrigerated fat from beef. Butter goes through a similar transition when it goes from cold to warm. The fat as it exists in the cuts of meat of beef and mutton or lamb is often called *suet.* Do you want to see what fat feels like? Shove your index finger (gently) into your belly just above your belly button. That's fat.

Have you ever seen a movie of surgery on the abdomen? The human fat layer you saw differed from fat on a cow only in that it was quite yellow, more like the color of the fat on chickens. When we speak of your "getting fat," we're talking about increasing the amount of this fatty or adipose tissue that you just poked with your finger. This fat layer can be present beneath the skin over virtually the whole body. It tends to be thinnest in places such as the soles of your feet and thickest around your middle.

Weight gain, therefore, generally means an increase in the amount of fat. Except in growing children, we don't gain weight by increasing the size of our bones or other connective tissue. It is possible to gain weight in your muscles, but this usually occurs only with a lot of "pumping iron."

If you are wondering why you were designed to so easily add more of this fat to your body, let me assure you that it truly serves a useful purpose beyond just providing you with a built-in seat cushion. We need to have some fat on our bodies. Although to most of us having less fat is better than having more, to have no fat would be undesirable to the point of being life threatening.

Fat's principal purpose is to serve as a storage depot for energy. There again is one of those words with multiple meanings, *energy*. We often use the word *energy* to mean pep or enthusiasm. When the country has an "energy crisis," it bears little relationship to your own lack of energy. We will generally use the word *energy* in this book to mean what physicist's understand by energy. It is what gives things the capacity to do work. Material substances can store energy. Oil and coal, for example, store energy. You are probably familiar with the various forms of energy: electricity, heat, light, etc. For the most part, one type can be converted into other types. Electrical energy is converted into light energy inside a light bulb. The energy stored inside your food, and later inside your body, is converted into heat energy to keep your body warm or is converted into mechanical energy that permits your muscles to pick up a heavy weight.

If it helps your understanding, consider energy as the useful component of fuel. Energy is what causes the wood in a fireplace to heat the room and what caused that sandwich at lunch to keep you working. All three classes of food substances—proteins, carbohydrates, and fats—supply energy, but fat holds more than twice as much energy per pound as do either of the other two. If it were possible for a person who has 30 pounds of excess fat on his body to store that energy in the form of protein or carbohydrate instead, he would weigh at least an extra 30 pounds. That's why, if you are going to store extra energy, it makes sense to store it as fat. In that way you will have less weight to carry around.

You've probably guessed that in the previous paragraphs, we could have substituted the word *calories* for the word *energy*. That's because calorie is one of the units of energy, specifically of heat energy. Because the amount of energy contained in food is generally determined by burning it in a special instrument, its energy content is best expressed in heat units, or calories.

Let's get back to the fat on your body. That's where you store the excess energy that is not immediately needed. You may ask, "Isn't it rather inefficient for me to carry my excess energy around with me wherever I go? Wouldn't it be more practical for me to store it in my refrigerator or my cupboard?" It might be more desirable to store your energy in those places, but it would probably create major problems if you needed some of this energy in a hurry and you couldn't get home.

As I discuss in later chapters, you are still this Stone Age character who has not yet adapted to the twenty-first century, and since that Paleolithic gent had no refrigerator or cupboard, you are not yet able to truly make full use of them either. When winter came or when times were otherwise tough, our ancestors should have been damn thankful for that same paunch that you now find so distasteful. For them, it is reasonable to assume that in many circumstances, the bigger the belly, the more chance there was for survival.

Fat is only the storage form of your fuel. The real fuel of your body is actually a type of sugar called *glucose*. It's a standard component of your blood, and there is a limited reserve supply in a somewhat different form in your liver, but when physical demands are made upon you and the supply is all used up, you must go to the energy bank to get more. That bank is the adipose tissue on your body. When needed, fat from your bank is converted into usable glucose. Be thankful the bank exists, but let's not keep too much of our energy in the bank account. It doesn't really pay much interest.

Do you like to eat fat? I've asked that question of thousands of patients over the years, except I phrased it differently. What I really asked was, "Do you eat a lot of fat?" The answer has been, almost without exception, "No, I don't like fat."

If I don't prompt my patient, I may get these kinds of elaborations:

"I always trim all the fat from my meat."
"I can't stand greasy foods."
"I never fry anything."
"I never use butter. Only margarine."
"I always use low-calorie margarine."
"I always broil my meat."
"I never fry chicken; I always bake it."

Since I'm not one to let sleeping dogs lie, I usually probe. It is then that I get a more complete picture. The lady who trims the visible fat from meat still eats plenty of meat and, thus, ingests considerable fat. The prudent guy who eats margarine doesn't realize that it has the same fat content as butter. The one who sticks to "diet" margarine is using a diluted fat, so in order to get the same satisfaction from it, he uses more of it, ending up with as much fat as if he had consumed the real stuff.

I love to ask about cheese. Almost everyone seems to like cheese. When I point out to my typical non-fat eaters that cheese contains a lot of fat, they appear surprised. Fat is deceptively present in many other foods. The concerned lady who coats her chicken with a dry, packaged product before she bakes it is usually stunned to learn that her oven-baked chicken ends up with about the same fat content as fried chicken. Nevertheless, she feels good about her baked chicken because she can say it isn't fried. In short, almost all of my patients eat a lot of fat. I must conclude that they really like it.

In the past 20 years or so, I have seen a proliferation of a type of restaurant that seems to be ever increasing in popularity. These are rather "cute," well run, theme restaurants, most of which have multiple franchise locations and specialize in "lighter" food. What is lighter is probably the price or the format. They are not fancy restaurants, but they have broad appeal. Their food comes to you looking very attractive, sometimes spectacular.

I have been with health-conscious people when they have ordered what they believed to be healthful selections. These are the kinds of people who don't eat meat or who use skim milk in their coffee. They order things such as "zucchini bonanza," which on casual glance appears to be squash slices heavily coated with a batter and deep fried. The thick coating or batter serves as a great sponge to soak up as much fat as possible from the deep fryer. But the food doesn't look greasy or fat. It is remarkably dry. These restaurant people are masters at hiding the fat. I guess that's why they are so successful. They may even serve the zucchini with some sort of a dip made with oil or perhaps melted cheese to up the fat content.

These same restaurants do similar things with lots of other foods. They serve us a ton of fat but make us comfortable by disguising it. They certainly know the formula for pleasing the public. To sum up the secret of their success, they serve very-high-fat food, and the public loves it. People stand in line for the opportunity to wolf down lots of fat. I don't think that the public is that naive. I believe that, in spite of the warnings about fat, they like it so much, they are willing to be taken in by the suggestion that these are not high-fat foods because they don't look like they are.

We have been conditioned. For as long as I can remember, it has not been fashionable to eat fat. We reflexively deny that we like fat, no matter how much of it we eat. To admit that you like fat is to admit to being out of step with the times.

I've traveled in the South, and I know to what extent lard and bacon grease are used to flavor dishes, particularly vegetable dishes. A true southern housewife must feel enormous guilt when she pours the bacon fat from her skillet down the drain. Did you ever eat "Red Eye Gravy"? I'm not going to give you the details of the recipe, but you start by using what's left after you have removed the bacon from the skillet.

What about this fixation with fat in the diet? Is this some sort of perverse or deviant behavior? If anything, not eating fat is deviant. Most of the world loves fat. The sauces that make French food French are loaded with fat. I don't know how my patients ever got the idea that Chinese or Thai food is low in fat. Have you ever watched an expert Chinese chef? Do you know how he keeps the food from sticking to his wok? He uses oil. He repeatedly adds oil at the first suggestion of sticking. And by the time you've eaten those eggrolls, the barbecued rib appetizer, and the chow mein, you're lubricated enough to slide out of the restaurant. Have you ever eaten only a Caesar salad because you were dieting? Ha! You may justify your love for Italian food by pointing out that they often use olive oil, but you are missing the point. Olive oil is fat just like butter is fat. Remember, I am not as yet discussing the relative merits of the various kinds of fat. I am simply pointing out that almost everyone loves fat.

Stefansson, the famous Arctic explorer (more about him in Chapter 10), reported that one of the great fears of the Eskimos with whom he lived for a time was fat deprivation. He said that when food was in short supply and they managed to kill an animal, if it was too lean, it did not solve their problem. The quest was always for game with a high fat content.

Isn't it ironic that this substance that we secretly adore as a food and the jellylike globs that cling to our bodies are really somewhat different forms of the same thing? We seem to have an inborn desire for the former and a congenital propensity to acquire the latter. It certainly makes it sound as if the general order of things is all screwed up. Wouldn't it make more sense if we were placed on Earth with an aversion to fatty foods and a predisposition to not store fat on our bodies?

Well, Nature is not all that insane. We have that need to store energy because we never know when the supply will be temporarily interrupted. And although we don't really need to eat fat to store it since our bodies are quite capable of converting both carbohydrates and proteins into stored fat, fat is still the most concentrated and practical way to acquire energy. If you are going on a long hike and you want to carry the minimum weight of high-energy provisions, you could carry a sack of sugar or a bottle of oil. Though neither alone is a good choice, to make my point, for the same energy value, you would need to carry only half the weight of oil.

The problem is that we are out of step with our times. Unless you are a homeless person who literally doesn't know where the next meal is coming from, you have little need to store much fat. If you fear another ice age, you will probably have ample warning and be given enough time to "fatten up." For the present, storing too much energy can be harmful, physically and psychologically, and it would be wise to divest yourself of your cache. But then, you already know that—that's why you're reading this book.

We should clear up the confusion over the names given to the various edible fats. I may mention *suet* from time to time in the book; it is simply the fat on the meat of cows or sheep. If we render (heat) suet, an oil is melted out of it, and if this oil is brought back to room temperature or refrigerated, it again becomes solid and is known as *tallow.* If we do the same thing to the fat removed from hogs, the resulting product is called *lard.*

*Oil* means fat that is a liquid at room temperature. Generally the oils used in cooking come from vegetable sources. *Grease* is an ill-defined term and is more descriptive of the appearance of substances rather than to identify them specifically. *Shortening* is a rather general term that could apply to almost any fat used as food. Bakers mix shortening with flour in order to "shorten" the finished product, making it softer and flakier.

Is there anything good we can say about the fat on our bodies, other than that it may save our lives if we are shipwrecked and have no food to eat? Is there anything positive that can be said for fat in our diet other that the suggestion that some vegetable or fish fats may actually protect against heart disease? We have already said that whether you admit it or not, it makes food more pleasurable. Its real value is that it *satisfies hunger.*

This is a totally ignored concept. It's not such a radical idea. It is actually well accepted. But it's not talked about. It is as though the nutritionists feel that to broadcast that information is akin to an endorsement of eating fat. This would not sit well in an age where fat is viewed as a four-letter word with only three letters. We have been programmed to think that, contrary to what seems to be our basic nature, fat is bad. But if you must eat it, then eat vegetable fats. But you shouldn't eat just any vegetable fat. "Tropical oils" are supposedly bad. Olive oil and canola oil are good. The general feeling is that you are supposed to get away from fat and switch to carbohydrate. Of course, the ultimate carbohydrate, sugar, is bad. The other carbohydrates, the "complex" ones, are good.

We have been following this advice for several years now. Dieters eat complex carbohydrates and count their fat grams. Athletes do the same and even "load" themselves with starch. For a while it was the national obsession.

Have you noticed that weight problems are not disappearing? The steady procession of my new overweight patients looks much the same as those of a few years ago or even 30 years ago. They still say the same things. Well, they say almost the same things. Years ago they would recite for me the list of diets that didn't work. Today they do the same, except they have new diets to disparage. They have been busy chomping on vegetables and hiding from fat in foods, and they are still overweight.

Over the years I've had experience with every pharmaceutical appetite depressant produced by man. Some drugs work fairly well but may have side effects. I will tell you what the best hunger suppressant that can be taken by mouth is. It's fat.

Yes, fat. Fat, of the three basic food substances, is by far the most satisfying of hunger. I can hear you saying, "So what? What good is it if it stops your hunger but gives you more calories than any other food? Isn't that like saying that the best way to kill your hunger is to eat a big eight-course meal?"

During the years that Stefansson spent on meat diets, he realized that a certain balance was necessary when mixing his protein (lean meat) with fat. If there were not enough fat, men would soon become weak and not be able to function. If they ate too much fat in relation to the amount of lean meat, they would become nauseated. Keep in mind that nausea is the extreme limit of hunger suppression. Have you ever eaten so much that you were on the brink of nausea? How was your appetite at that moment? Appetite and nausea don't coexist. Have you ever crossed the line and actually achieved real nausea? At that moment the last thing you wanted was food.

In the back of your mind, are you troubled by all this talk of fat, particularly animal fat, in the diet? The question of safety has to be bugging you. Isn't eating fat associated with cholesterol, and isn't that a bad idea?

Fat controls hunger. Physiology books tell us that one way it does so is by slowing down the emptying time of the stomach. It is not useful to look into the various reasons that it works in the scope of this book. Suffice it to say that it is a generally recognized principle that fat satisfies hunger. But in today's world, as an adjunct to weight loss, it is never considered. That has not always been the case.

When I was first in practice in the late fifties and into the sixties, I had a certain number of patients who would recount their successes on various diets that they got from best-selling books. I was not too long out of school, and I naively believed almost everything I had been told by my professors. They were generally negative about most diet programs. The word was that people should control their weights through strength of character and personal discipline. I had also kept up with the literature and subscribed to numerous professional journals. No sooner would one diet book appear than scathing criticism in the scientific media would tear it apart. Followers of Dr. Stillman's diet or Dr. Atkins' diet or Dr. Taller's diet were told that they must get off those meat-centric diets or they would die. As I look back, I suspect the mortality rate of obese people was far higher than the death rate of those following the various diets. In fact, I never heard of a documented death directly attributable to any of those diets.

So when one patient after another came to me and told me that they had done just great on one of the meat or meat-fat diets, I would shrug it off and tell them they were lucky to be alive and I would proceed with more mainstream methods. It took a lot of years in practice before I really took a second look at what was not mainstream thinking but nevertheless seemed promising.

We will examine a number of these diets in detail in Chapter 11. There were more of them than you might think. Each had its quirks and gimmicks. All were high protein. Some were high fat also. The public liked these diets, followed them, bought the books that espoused them, and lost weight. But the dieters were also exposed to the barrage of criticism and reports of the ominous effects of following such diets, and in the end, they faded in popularity, only to be replaced by alternative methods that produced poorer results.

To sum up, I know that we can lose weight comfortably by eating diets very high in protein and low in carbohydrate. We can even lose weight, in some circumstances, on diets high in fat. There is, however, real question as to the safety of such systems given what we have been told about cholesterol and fat.

The overweight problem is so serious and widespread that nothing that offers a glimmer of hope should be ignored. We cannot summarily dismiss the success of these diets simply because some "experts" brand them unacceptable. Even if there is some merit to the warnings, perhaps there are positive elements of these diets that can be preserved, while the negative elements are modified.

*Chapter 7*

# What Is Meat?

I've used up a lot of hours discussing food with my patients. Well, why not? That's what it's all about, isn't it? Haven't they come to visit me because of food?

At times I am impressed by the depth of knowledge that my patients have about certain aspects of food. If I spend time with them, I come away learning something. At other times, I'm shocked by how ignorant some of us are regarding the nature of the stuff we put into our stomachs. This is particularly true when it comes to meat.

Any discussion of food must inevitably include meat. It's always a shock when I realize that the person across the desk from me truly does not understand what meat is. Usually I discover this only after I've said something such as, "Animal muscle is a rich source of protein." This seems like a rather obvious statement.

The patient might counter with, "I never eat muscle," and I immediately see that she really doesn't understand about meat. In the United States, where I live, beef, chicken, pork, turkey, lamb, fish, and seafood are the most popular kinds of meat. For the moment let's confine the discussion to beef, although much of what I say will apply to the others as well. For my explanation,

I've chosen one of the mammals—cows—because their meat is somewhat like our meat.

Like us, they are made up of a variety of different materials, or "tissues." They have skin and bones, which we do eat but in a limited and disguised way. Cattle have organs such as the liver, kidney, brain, pancreas, and the like and we do eat these parts, but most people do not consider them as mainstream when it comes to eating meat.

What we generally picture when the discussion turns to meat are such old standbys as sizzling steaks, rare roast beef, monster drive-in hamburgers, smoky beef ribs, etc. From what tissues of the animal do these cuts come? Is it possible you don't know that they're principally muscle? When we say "meat," we usually mean muscle. It's not all muscle, but it's mostly muscle. Mixed in is undoubtedly a fair amount of fat, some thin membrane called fascia, and many small blood vessels, most of which go unnoticed. There may be some other things such as pieces of nerves, tendons, or ligaments, that are really tough and that we'll generally leave on the plate. The important thing is that when we talk of eating meat, we're generally talking about muscle.

It's muscle that allows cows and humans and all other animals to move. For the most part, plant foods can't move. That could be considered one of the distinguishing elements that separate plants from animals. We move by contracting (shortening) particular groups of muscles. When a muscle shortens, it usually pulls a bone one way or the other. Every time you scratch your back, lots of muscles are moving lots of bones around. Muscle shortening accounts for how cows and humans walk. When we talk, we do so by contracting certain muscles of our faces, necks, and chests. And when you blink, tiny muscles are at work.

Does it seem logical that the best food for building or repairing our own human muscles (our meat) might be the food that is most similar to our own muscles? I think that sounds logical, but that doesn't necessarily make it true. Don't accept that yet.

Some of my patients don't eat meat. At least they say that they don't eat meat. What's more, they often say it with a kind of a flourish. Sometimes they alert me to this fact for no other reason than to be informative. More often it is flaunted as though it were an accomplishment for which one should be proud. At any rate, it usually comes out early in our relationship. I don't have to ask. They all seem to use exactly the same words. They simply say, "I don't eat meat."

If I probe, and I usually do, I learn that they truly don't make a clear distinction between eating food of animal origin and that from plants. Their vegetarian principles have often been compromised to satisfy their own particular needs or philosophies. They might say such things as, "I've never really liked meat," but it is more likely that they will attach some moral or religious significance to their choice of diet.

They might say that they don't eat meat because it's unhealthful, and the discussion might then go on to cholesterol and fat. Or they might say that they consider it wrong to kill animals just for one's own eating pleasure. I'm pretty well prepared to counter that one. If they tell me that they don't eat meat because their religion forbids it, the discussion usually ends right there. What more can one say?

There are various possible interpretations of the statement *I don't eat meat.* It could mean that they don't eat beef, pork, or lamb but they do eat chicken or turkey or fish. I won't bore you with the tortured thinking that produces that set of rules. Others don't eat meat but will eat things derived from or removed from animals. For example, they do eat butter, milk, eggs, etc. It's not unlike me to inquire thus, "Do you know that the cake you had last night was probably made with butter that came from milk that was pumped out of a cow?"

I like to ask the more smug among them if they eat gelatin. Can you think of anything that appears less meatlike than a bowl of raspberry gelatin? They surely know the origins of gelatin. Some eat it; others don't.

Some of my patients are dedicated vegetarians. They not only do *not eat meat*, but they are on a mission, hell-bent on converting the rest of us. They are well armed with arguments passed down to them, contentions that they've rehearsed and refined. The subject might move on to the dangers of meat, the immorality of it, and maybe even of the basic nature of man. They say that we obviously were not intended to eat meat. We are not constructed like other meat-eating animals. We don't have sharp teeth for killing our prey and tearing meat, as do tigers and wolves. We don't have claws, but rather flat fingernails, which are better suited for picking berries and opening nuts, similar to those of chimpanzees and baboons, animals who they incorrectly believe don't eat meat.

The more avid among them may even go into dissertations on the biochemistry of our bodies or the comparative anatomy of digestive systems, but of late I cut short the instructional sessions because I usually have other patients waiting. To sum up, when it comes to eating meat, I hear everything from interesting arguments to utter drivel.

Well, what about meat? Should we eat it or shouldn't we? Should we eat a lot of it or perhaps only a little? In making this decision, to whom should we listen? Should we rely solely on the latest dicta from the scientific community presumably passed down to us by the media, or should we become scholars and survey the whole question from a historical perspective?

I've personally done it all. That's my job. For the moment let's examine the latter alternative.

Without a doubt the most confusing bit of jargon that has been added to our vocabularies is the word *natural*. It's the buzz word that gained prominence in the eighties and nineties and decided to try to stay with us forever. God forbid! "Is it natural?" I'm asked. It can apply to food, medications, exercise, even attitudes. It always floors me because I must be honest with you, I don't know what's natural.

I can't make a quick trip to the supermarket without spotting the word dozens of times. It shares top billing with the phrases such as *no cholesterol* and *no trans fats.* But what is natural? For that matter, what is unnatural? Or is that the opposite of natural? Maybe the opposite of natural is supernatural.

Most often my patients apply the word to foods. They seem to hint that if you alter the food in any way from how it exists in nature, then it is no longer natural. But it's impractical not to alter it. I can't picture any of my patients eating wheat or corn right from the stalk while it's still growing. That sounds pretty natural, but I prefer my corn boiled and my wheat baked. You have to alter them. The crops have to be harvested. That's a form of alteration. And it's usually done by monstrous machines. Does that render them not natural?

If you grind the wheat, does it lose its claim to being natural? If you remove the outer shell, the bran, or perhaps the wheat germ, is it no longer natural? If you then take that nice, white powder that you get when you grind wheat, and mix it with water and yeast, then let it stand, and finally heat it in an oven where it puffs up to three times its original size, do you still have something natural? Is bread natural?

When we give an orange a very unnatural squeeze, is the stuff that comes out of it natural? When a squirrel alters a nut by removing the shell, is that natural? Do we change the natural quality of things simply by altering them?

The proponents of the natural generally classify "chemicals" as not natural. They don't seem to recognize that everything in our world is chemical. Your own body is a complicated mixture of chemicals. Earth is one big chemical laboratory. When we produce food, we chop it, grind it, mix it with other foods, and heat it in various ways. That's the same kind of thing that they do when they make plastic or tires or aspirin. They start with materials that either grow or are dug from the earth and they grind them and heat them and mix them until they get the substance they want.

My own view is that if it is something that has its origins in the brain of man, it's natural. If it's produced by scheming, invisible demons, then it's unnatural.

What, then, is the natural food of man? There's a question for you! What type of food were we intended to eat? Did I say intended? By whom? By God? By Nature? Let's try to understand this business of natural. We all know that tigers eat other animals and cows eat grass and grains and we regard those diets as natural for them. It is their usual diet; it is what tigers and cows have always eaten. What, then, is the natural diet of man?

If we look to the Bible, we get a rather mixed answer. A lot of food is mentioned in the Bible, but it seems to be about the same general mix that we eat today: bread, milk, meat, wine, eggs, fruit, vegetables, etc.

At the beginning of Genesis, God seems to have prescribed the diet for Adam and Eve. According to the King James version, God said, "I have given you every herb bearing seed, which is upon the face of all the earth, and every tree, in the which is the fruit of the tree yielding seed; to you it shall be for meat. And it was so."

I am hardly a biblical scholar, but it would seem to me that Adam and Eve were instructed that they are to eat fruits and vegetables and that it is as good as meat. Or you could interpret this to mean that things that grow are an adequate substitute for meat. Still, meat must be desirable in some way. Why else would you need to substitute something for it?

After the big flood, the rules seemed to have changed. Noah emerged from the arc with these instructions from God:

> *Every moving thing that liveth shall be meat for you; even as the green herb have I given you all things.*

If my interpretation is correct, man is now instructed to add meat to his list. It is logical to believe that immediately after a major flood, there wouldn't be too much edible vegetation. Were the animals that were sheltered in the arc intended to be breeding stock for the future subsistence of man?

I leave the Bible for those who spend their lives deciphering it, but I will point out that it does not seem to prescribe vegetarianism.

The scientific world perhaps holds clearer clues. Scientists tell us that this planet upon which we stand has been around for a long time. As a child, I remember reading a fanciful view of the history of the world. I think it was an article in *Reader's Digest,* but I'm not certain. The writer asked us to view the history of the world as a lengthy movie that took a full year to view in its entirety. That single year would be a proportional condensation of the world from the time it was created until the then present time. He described what was happening as the movie progressed from the world's beginnings on January 1 to the last second of December 31, which was the current time. Much of the year was taken up with the hot ball cooling down. As I recall, it said that life did not appear until sometime in December and that man made his first appearance *in the last five minutes of the very last day of the year.* All that the human race has accomplished, from our prehistoric origins to our invention of pizza and Bluetooth headsets, took place in the last few seconds of those last five minutes. This still impresses me, though not enough to make me get out my pocket calculator to verify his figures. It does tend to put our presence and importance in the scheme of things into a more modest perspective.

Biblical scholars have tried to date the planet by analysis of the ages of biblical characters and other clues from the text. That's rough going; you have to make a lot of smart guesses.

*And Re'u lived two and thirty years, and begat Se'rug:*

*And Re'u lived after he begat Se'rug two hundred and seven years, and begat sons and daughters.*

*And Se'rug lived thirty years, and begat Ne'hor:*

*And Se'rug lived after he begat Ne'hor two hundred years, and begat sons and daughters.*

Aside from wondering what diet Re'u and Se'rug followed to achieve such longevity, I find this type of calculation tedious. Understandably, there has been a lot of variation in the estimates. One scholar said the world was created in 4004 B.C., another in 3928 B.C. Another felt that the above-mentioned flood was in 2349 B.C. The Hebrew calendar supposedly starts with creation and puts that event at less than 6,000 years ago.

Scientists believe that it has been somewhat longer. The most recent estimates suggest that Earth came into existence almost 4 billion years ago. That's more than a half million times as long as any of the above estimates.

One thing seems certain: one of the most curious of the organisms that populated Earth, and perhaps one of the most complicated, was certainly a long time in coming. According to the scientists, by the time man arrived, Earth was very old indeed.

Why do you marvel at ancient structures that might be more than 1,000 years old? Your own home was built on a piece of property that might be 4 billion years old.

By now you should have a sense that man has been preoccupied with meat for a very long time. In the next three chapters we'll explore the critical role of meat in the evolution of the human race.

Chapter 8

# Chapter 8

# Meat Has Always
# Been the Way

I have learned during my 50-plus years of treating overweight patients that the best diet for losing weight is one that contains a lot of protein and much less carbohydrate.

If you are as old as I am or even 20 or so years younger, you can probably remember when losing weight was not all that complicated. You would simply concentrate on eating the meat of cattle, fowl, or fish and keep away from starches such as bread and potatoes, and you could reasonably expect the weight to fall off your body. That was in the era when *cholesterol* was some poorly understood term (as if that were no longer true) and fats were not categorized as good or evil.

So what happened? The terms *complex carbohydrates*, and *net carbs*, and *fat grams* hadn't been invented yet. Consequently we simply went on what was called a high-protein, low-carbohydrate diet and we lost weight. Perhaps we did it with help. Maybe there was a book by Dr. Stillman or Dr. Atkins in the picture. Or perhaps the family doctor had a hand in it. Reducing didn't seem that difficult. Everyone knew how to lose weight.

But something happened. We forgot about the diets that worked or we were frightened away from them. By the 1980s we were introduced to the new nemesis of the human race, cholesterol, and in a flash, meat became as undesirable as toxic waste and losing weight suddenly became both complex and difficult.

Of course, this new insight was not all bad. It spawned new industries, many of which prospered. Jobs were created. Packaged meals with attractive pictures on the cartons were purchased by the millions, and the advertising people had a field day promoting new weight-loss schemes. New job titles such as "nutritional counselor" and "personal trainer" were created. In the process, weight loss became a national obsession.

Frightened away from losing weight the old-fashioned way, we discovered that the pounds didn't come off very easily with these new, supposedly more healthful theories. The great overweight public looked for help. They, of course, had no trouble finding it. Weight-loss helpers sprang up overnight like mushrooms. Anyone with enough dollars could buy a weight-loss franchise and reap the benefits of nationwide advertising. If you wanted to get into the reducing business, you would pay your money and, with a two-day seminar, they would turn you into an expert not only in weight loss, but also in such diverse skills as selecting waiting room furniture or pressuring a desperate client into buying a course of treatment.

Not all the purveyors of weight-loss wisdom installed themselves in plush quarters. Some set up shop literally on the street. Badges that invited us to query the wearer on how to lose weight were worn by hordes of nondescript individuals we encountered in the course of our meandering. It didn't matter that these badge-bearers had no diplomas on their walls; they had no walls. It didn't even matter that these advice-givers might not have received kindergarten educations, let alone education in proper nutrition. Were you to have asked them how to lose weight, you would have been told the secret. Not only that, you would have been invited to wear a badge and tell other people how to lose weight. You could have thus become part of a gigantic pyramid of weight-loss experts who were dedicated to making the expert at the apex very rich indeed.

Yet we all knew that they, like many others with a variety of dubious schemes, were fringe operators, and even though, as a lark, we might patronize them, we had more respect for those counselors whose advice made it into the conventional literature. If a popular magazine of the nineties talked of high intake of complex carbohydrates, we accepted it as gospel. If some familiar entertainment figure held court on the television airwaves and railed against fat grams, who were we to dispute such authority?

Of the many systems that I could construct to classify my patients, the one that might be most relevant to this discussion would be to position them by their ages. It boils down to two groups. The older ones remember how weight loss used to be and freely show their discomfort with the new theories or at least express a kind of nostalgic recollection of the old ways. Then there are the younger folks who seem to be oblivious to the knowledge that there was ever any other way.

The truth is that the rather recent frenzy for eating the right kind of carbohydrates as a means of becoming beautiful and slim, while viewing meat as some sort of environmental poison, seemed to be a new national preoccupation.

If you are part of the younger group, it won't take much research on your part to learn that my pronouncements are not original at all. What I have been telling you had been the opinion not only shared by the public for many years, but also of the "experts," those who ministered to the public, those who wrote the books, those doctors whose advice we all respected. The notion that you can lose weight by eating potatoes and grains and pasta would have been a bizarre departure from reason. A few short years back, that's the diet you would have followed if you had wanted to *gain* weight. To lose weight, you would have eaten protein—meat.

Even at this early stage, you probably have an inkling of what I will be proposing in the pages to come, and it is only logical that you should be thinking something such as this:

"Suppose he's right. What difference does it make? I'm not about to go on an all-meat diet. We all hear that meat is unhealthy and maybe even dangerous. I want to lose weight, but I don't want to kill myself in the process."

I certainly can't find fault with these musings. For quite some time, you have been fed a steady stream of information that assigns certain words to the list of ingestible things to be avoided by prudent individuals—*meat, cholesterol, fat, food dyes, hormones,* and the like. Some of these warnings have merit; others may not be as valid.

This book is not an exhaustive treatise on nutrition. I have confined my words and advice to that subject that occupies the better part of each of my days, the means of achieving a healthful weight by a safe method. I've tried not to bore you with nutritional pseudo-wisdom. I haven't said much about subjects not directly related to your weight. I am going to tell you how to lose weight comfortably, quickly, and safely. It will be necessary for you to ignore some of the current nonsense with which you have been bombarded. I will be advocating the kind of diet that works, that has always worked, and that is the most natural for us humans.

To that information, I'm going to add a new element—the way to ease your hunger while you're eating the right diet. You already know that the word *cookie* is going to play an important part.

If you think that the produce section of the supermarket contains the foods that are the most appropriate for the human animal, let me instruct you that fruits and vegetables are the "new" foods of our upright species. Man just started eating these about 10,000 years ago. That's like yesterday in comparison to the time that our ancestors have been roaming the earth. And being nomadic, they really did roam. In those days, you had to be on the move if you hoped to find meat. You can't grow fruits and vegetables if you don't stay in one place. During the rest of those years that man has existed, he ate meat with some occasional fruits, nuts, or berries if he could find them. But he craved meat. He probably spent every waking hour searching for meat. He thrived on meat. Our ancestors survived on meat.

What's more, you exist because they were able to find meat and did survive. It's not too early in this book for you to begin to ask yourself these questions:

If meat is such bad food for us humans, how did our ancestors survive millions of years of eating virtually nothing but meat? Isn't my own existence the result of the human race's successful battle for survival?

This kind of thinking must inevitably turn to the consideration of that demon that today haunts our health-oriented literature: cholesterol. What about cholesterol? Is it not dangerous? Is meat not full of it?

The answer to the last question is a clear yes. The meat you eat contains cholesterol and so does the meat on your own body. The answer about the danger of eating cholesterol is not as clear. There is a real diversity of opinion about the cholesterol thing. Not all scientists believe that you are getting correct information about this subject. The more extreme critics of the current widespread campaign against cholesterol call it a money-making scam foisted upon the public. I don't know about its being a scam, but I can tell you that it is making money for certain people. The public's fear of cholesterol in the bloodstream has been a windfall to the medical, drug, and food industries.

Getting back to losing weight, I consider myself to be a student of that subject. I'm really fascinated by the complexities of man's search for slimness and the difficulty of achieving it. I even collect diet books with the hope that collective wisdom of the past may be of value in solving some of these mysteries. The authors in my library go far beyond such familiar names as Atkins, Agatston, and Sears. Have you forgotten Dr. Irwin Maxwell Stillman? His books sold millions. He said that you lose weight by eating meat. Dr. Herman Taller's advice? Eat meat.

More recently, Dr. Atkins wrote some books. He said you lose weight by eating meat. A lot of people have followed his advice over the years. If anything, the most recent trend seems to be to get back to eating meat.

If you think that I have selected a few mavericks from the ranks of the other rational weight-loss experts, you are incorrect. You're going to hear about quite a few more.

The authors of the most recent books that allow meat are written by the better-known names, the more flamboyant. Over the years there have been a slew of others who have held the same view. The chances are that you have not heard of Donaldson, Mackarness, or Pennington. They were less sensational yet perhaps even more respected. They all offered the same general advice: high protein, meat.

You might have heard of Banting. He was the nineteenth-century man who possibly started it all. He was so pleased with the meat diet that his doctor gave him, the diet that helped him lose weight, that in 1863 he wrote a book about it and gave it away. A lot of other writers quote Banting. We will certainly talk more about "Bantingism."

These experts and many more like them didn't do much hemming and hawing. They weren't shy. They told it like it was. One of them was Blake Donaldson, a New York physician who was then the respected guru of weight loss. He was the one who knowledgeable New Yorkers flocked to in order to get thin. Hold on to your hats, folks. Here is an excerpt from the instructions he gave his patients in 1962:

*You are going to lose weight, while rebuilding the cells in your arteries with something called amino acids, so I want you to get about at least one half pound of any fresh meat you like with each meal. Shell steak with fat on it, two double ribbed Frenched lamb chops, club cuts of roast beef one half inch thick, or home chopped meat with suet in it seem the best.*

Here is how Alfred William Pennington, MD, who ran the obesity program for E. I. DuPont de Nemours & Co., the chemical giant, put it in a 1953 paper he wrote for *The Journal of Clinical Nutrition:*

**First course of each meal:** *One half-pound or more of fresh meat with the fat. This part of the diet is unlimited. You can eat as much as you want. The proper proportion is three parts lean to one part fat. Most of the meat you buy is not fat enough, so get extra beef kidney fat, slice it and fry it to make up the proper proportion. Good meats are roast beef, steak, roast lamb, lamb chops, stewed beef, fresh pork, and pork chops. Hamburger is all right if you grind it yourself just before it is cooked.*

When *Holiday* magazine (it's gone now but was very popular in its day) got wind of Pennington's diet and published it, it was picked up by thousands, and the public response was so enthusiastic that the magazine continued to resurrect it for years.

Let's stop right here and regroup. This advice didn't come from Dr. Siegal. These quotes came from Blake Donaldson and Alfred Pennington. We can't question these good doctors about it because they have departed. Blake's patients followed his advice and lost a ton of weight. Pennington probably reduced hundreds who worked for DuPont before the public embraced it and the numbers skyrocketed. I haven't given you my dietary advice yet, but I do urge you to read on until I do.

The idea that high-protein diets were *the* way to lose weight was not simply the secret knowledge of a select group of savants. Everyone knew this. This information was public property. When I first went into medical practice in 1957, no one thought that there was any other way.

The enthusiasm for meat didn't come from just doctors. The great Arctic explorer Stefansson wrote extensively and eloquently whole volumes on the virtues of eating meat, and what's more, eating meat exclusively. His fervor was based on years of living with Eskimos and sharing with them what he felt was the perfect diet for the human race. He liked to call it the Stone Age Diet, and other writers have picked up on the name. Not too long ago, Stefansson's widow assured me that, as a result of his meat diet, "Stef" enjoyed perfect health. I might add, Stefansson didn't eat just meat, he ate *fatty* meat.

I hope this introduction stimulates your curiosity. I have just touched on the subject. Don't rush out and buy that cow just yet. You really don't have enough information to make any decisions based on the words of Donaldson, Pennington, or Stefansson. Let's learn from them, but let's use this knowledge to lose weight safely. Don't try yet. Be patient. Let's take the time to really understand what weight loss is all about. I am going to build my case for the diet that works, the diet that has always worked, the diet that will make you thin.

*Chapter 9*

# Our Carnivorous Ancestors

D oesn't it seem like we are deluged with information and instructions from self-proclaimed experts as to what we should eat, not only to get or stay thin, but also to be healthy in general? Those who pass on this advice, not too sheepishly, suggest that they know the answer. But do they really? Did you ever wonder how they came by such important knowledge? I'm still wondering.

Would knowing what our distant ancestors ate offer some clues as to what's the optimal diet for man? Obviously, enough of our very distant relatives survived on what they ate or I wouldn't be writing and you wouldn't be reading these words. So what did they eat?

The food they ate wasn't procured from supermarkets, nor was it prepared from cookbooks authored by celebrity chefs. Anthropologists seem to have made some pretty good guesses as to the diet of early man. Scientists at least offer some measure of proof as a basis for their conclusions. They tell us that our distant relatives, those with names like Cro-magnon and *Homo neander-thalensis*, were not really that different from us. Sure, 100,000 to 200,000 years have passed since they were around, but considering how long other living organisms have inhabited our planet, in the scheme of things, the first appearance of humans was really not that long ago.

What many or these scientists have concluded is that the foods our ancestors ate that enabled them to survive might be just as useful to us. The point is that not enough time has gone by for us to have adapted to a different type of diet, the type now available to us.

The important thing to remember is that we as a species have not changed much physically in those past 100,000 years. We are still the same organism. Our arms, legs, backbones, stomachs, livers, and brains are essentially the same. Likewise, physiological functions and chemical processes that take place inside our bodies have probably changed little over the years. This includes how we digest and use food.

A 1992 article in *The Journal of Public Health* attempted to explain how we have not yet defined exactly what we humans should eat. Rather than speak of the normal human diet, it talks of the "optimal" diet. The authors, borrowing this knowledge from others before them, take notice of this point:

> *Meanwhile, the physiologic processes in the human body most likely have not changed or adapted biologically for thousands, perhaps hundreds of thousands, of years. Our metabolic processes are no different from those of our prehistoric ancestors, determined largely by their existing environment.*

Though our brain hasn't changed functionally, what we put into that brain has clearly changed. The brain, along with its other functions, is a repository for information. It is analogous to the hard disk on your personal computer, but its storage capacity is enormous. It also contains the rest of the guts of your personal computer, so it is able to process the information. It does everything your computer does and then some. Its only failing is that in most cases it is considerably slower than your computer.

Alvin Toffler, in his 1970 book, *Future Shock,* tells us that our scientific knowledge, as reflected in the numbers of articles in scientific journals, doubles every 15 years. That means that we now have perhaps six or seven times as much scientific knowledge as when he wrote his book. This is awesome to contemplate. If you work backward using the corollary that as you go back in time, for each 15 years the sum total of knowledge is cut in half, by the time you reach 4 million years ago, you must come to the conclusion that although early man had our same large brain, his was practically empty. There just wasn't much data to store. That's not surprising. The purpose of all those scientific papers is to communicate the information to others. In early times, the only knowledge that could have been acquired from other members of your own species would have been from those with whom you had actual contact since knowledge wasn't recorded on paper or electronically. That's why our ancestors didn't know very much.

In terms of diet, they probably hadn't yet learned how to make dishes like lasagna, although later they did acquire some mastery of fire, so I'm not going to rule out their version of prime rib. I'm not trying to be flippant, but I do want to drive home the point that in terms of progress, things move very slowly when the brain has little knowledge with which to work. They probably were intelligent enough, but they lacked information. Their primitive tools were not much more than rocks with a few chips taken out of them, and those devices would remain unchanged for thousands of years. Compare that with the certainty that the complicated appliance you just bought will be obsolete in five years.

Eating is automatic. When we're hungry, we just do it; no one has to remind us. That's a good thing. Without hunger, some of us might forget to eat and would, consequently, starve to death. When our brains tell us we're hungry, we go out and look for food. Our ancient ancestors did the same thing. In fact, it's probable that looking for food was their chief occupation. Remember, there was no backup system in those days, no convenience store to run to when they were out of food. If they were to survive, they needed to find food.

Anthropologists generally refer to these people as hunter-gatherers. Their emphasis is usually on the hunter part. The main pursuit was hunting; gathering probably took place in a more hit-and-miss fashion as an adjunct to the former.

A lot of books have been written on man as a hunter. Many suggest that our predatory predilection is actually instinctual. Ask the National Rifle Association what they think about limiting our access to the tools of hunting. Some cultural anthropologists have interpreted the fact that men kill other men today as a natural consequence of our basic nature and our love of the hunt.

One of the better authors on this subject was Robert Ardrey. He was primarily a writer of plays and Hollywood films, but his true love was anthropology and ethology, and he devoted years to research in those fields. Between 1961 and 1976, he wrote four books on the subject of the origins of man's basic nature. He talked with the foremost researchers of his time. Ardrey gives the impression of both loving and hating the human race. His first nonfiction book, *African Genesis,* was sort of an homage to Raymond Dart, who made a most important discovery, the bones of a specimen who lived 4 to 5 million years ago in Africa and whom Dart named *Australopithecus africanus.*

Dart was convinced that his Australopithecus was both a tool maker and big game hunter. His find broke new ground, for it moved man's origins from Asia to Africa and emphasized our hunting nature. His paper that followed, "The Predatory Nature of Man," was not well received. It rocked the boat. Only most recently have his findings become more widely accepted.

By the time Robert Ardrey had written his fourth nonfiction book, *The Hunting Hypothesis,* he seemed to have clearly developed his thesis:

> *Man is man, and not a chimpanzee, because for millions upon millions of evolving years we killed for a living.*

Ardrey believed that for perhaps a few hundred thousand years our ancestors depended on killing to survive. Because of our "big brain" and our inventive nature, we were able to do it well, perhaps surpassing all other animals in that skill.

Not everyone agreed, but Ardrey furnished his evidence, and it was difficult to refute. His critics were armed more with rhetoric than with solid evidence. His friend, Louis Leakey, one of the most famous anthropologists at the time, was not as certain as Ardrey that man had been such a great hunter. There was no dispute that he was a carnivore, a meat-eater, but Leakey leaned toward the notion that man got his meat by settling for "road kill," by being a scavenger. In other words, he felt that early man was more inclined to let other animals do his dirty work, the kill, and that he simply took the leftovers.

Ardrey disagreed. He didn't believe that man could sustain life that way. He felt if man had the guts to steal food from fierce beasts, he had the courage to go after his own prey. In a debate with Louis Leakey, reprinted in *Psychology Today* in 1972, Ardrey makes his point:

> *If we go back 500,000 years to* Homo sapiens, *the big-brained man, there isn't much question about what went on. They were definitely hunters. This heritage has had a tremendous effect upon us in terms of natural selection. Those men who had an efficient capacity for violence, who enjoyed violence, were the men who survived and passed on their genes. If you didn't like to go out and hunt, you*

*wouldn't get the girl, and you wouldn't get any food—you'd
just be an extra mouth to feed. And I would assert that we
didn't live off of spinach. This is a fashionable point of view
much promoted in American anthropology. Lettuce is great
for diets, but not for men who have to work for a living. We
had to live off meat.*

Ardrey's estimate of *Homo sapiens* arrival at a half million years
ago was over twice that of current thinking. It is generally accepted
that from 150,000 to 200,000 years ago, *Homo sapiens* did hunt
animals. He got his meat by killing, and he was good at it.

Dr. Lyall Watson independently developed similar ideas but
with some differences. Watson, a South African zoologist and
a director of the Johannesburg Zoo, shared Ardrey's opinion
of the killing nature of early man. In his book *The Omnivorous
Ape*, he states:

*Man is what he is and does what he does because he once
was a killer. He was hungry and needed food, and the food
he most wanted was meat. So he applied his growing brain to
the problem of killing—and started a chain of circumstances
that still affects our lives today. Because our ancestors needed
greater speed, they became more upright and today we have
vertical men. Because they needed artificial weapons, tools
were developed and today we have elaborate instrumenta-
tion. Because cooperation was essential, their brains became
even more complex, and a language and a culture came into
being. Today we also have spinal disorders, ballistic missiles
and racial disturbances, but we have had to take the bad
with the good. Both were produced by our diet.*

Notice that Watson seems to be saying that man "was" a killer.
That should make a lot of people a lot more comfortable though
they'll probably still lock their doors at night. He obviously differs

from Ardrey in that he believes that we have channeled that aggressive nature into more socially acceptable directions.

> *Man relinquished his role as a killer and hunter when he became a settled farmer about 10,000 years ago. He became domesticated and well fed, but he still needed to hunt. . . . In a million years of hunting, man formed close ties with other adult males in the tribe and grew used to a life involving constant risks and challenges. So he turned work into an activity that involved him, with other men, in a recurring gamble that has many characteristics of the hunt. To take an example from only one kind of work (business centers) where the prey (his rivals) could be stalked (with the aid of industrial espionage) and captured (in a take-over bid).*

I don't know if the question of whether *Homo sapiens* started out a great hunter or gradually acquired his hunting skills over time will ever be settled. Is the killer instinct still with him? I don't know that either, but we can leave that subject now. Our interest is in what he ate and how well he fared on essentially the same diet for hundreds of thousands of years. The diet was mostly meat. The acquisition of meat occupied his thoughts and time. Depending on where he lived and the seasonal climatic changes, failing to find meat was to face death. Meat was serious stuff. But in the end, he obviously did a good job of keeping himself supplied because he lasted until the Agricultural Revolution, an event that began just yesterday.

Most authorities put man's entry into farming at between 8,000 and 13,000 years ago. Remember how slowly things moved back then. A hundred generations would go by with little to no change in farming techniques. Some experts feel that although man farmed, he really didn't get his act together until about 5,000 years ago.

Remember that movie I spoke about, the one where the history of our earth was crowded into a single year? The Agricultural Revolution started well into the last minute of that year. If you didn't have an accurate enough stopwatch, you would have to say that agriculture, the birth of Christ, the U.S. Civil War, and Google all occurred at about the same instant. My poor attempt at humor is only meant to drive home the point that we have just this minute discovered the fruits of the harvest after countless lifetimes of eating meat. Food that grows is like a new gadget that you just purchased. You don't even know how to use it yet.

If you didn't know it before, by now it should be rather clear to you that all of our ancestors existed on meat. Was that their complete diet? Probably not. They likely also ate nuts, berries, maybe roots, and whatever else they could find. But principally they ate meat. They didn't seem to be in a hurry to get away from meat-eating, although eventually they did begin to add more and more plant foods.

By contrast, the ancestors of our ancestors, the ones who didn't particularly look like us, were probably mostly vegetarians. That's why physically those earliest folks had many of the physical characteristics of other principally vegetarian primates (such as apes). Obviously, the supply of food such as nuts and berries was not as reliable as when a group of men working together were able to corner and kill a large animal. This could supply a number of people with food for days.

The major event that precipitated our movement away from plant foods was probably the drought that afflicted Africa for some 12 million years. Have you ever experienced a heat wave that lasted a whole month? Can you imagine a climatic disaster that lasted for 12 million years? It was probably the major stimulus for adaptation. So here we have this paradox. Here is an animal that physically appears to be designed to eat plants, but because he has a brain that is capable of reasoning and invention, no matter how primitive, he has discovered that he can survive better by eating meat.

That is exactly what he did. He ate meat. There is little controversy on this point. Anthropologists argue about whether he actually did the hunting or used other hunting animals' leftovers, but there is no doubt that he lived on meat. He probably did so for some 3 million years. During that time the process of natural selection was operative just as it is today. Those individuals for whom meat-eating was not the optimal diet may have perished. Those mutants for whom meat-eating was ideal survived, reproduced, and eventually produced guess who? You!

That is why *you are they and they are you.*

It appears that these early people followed the herd, so to speak. Some scientists believe that they probably worked in large groups. Their techniques are well documented by their art on the walls of caves. They were essentially nomadic. They followed the food, and since the food moved, so did they.

It wasn't until about 10,000 years ago that they finally settled down. They established permanent or semi-permanent homes for themselves. What changed the whole picture was agriculture. A new lifestyle was in order. Since crops stay put, man had to settle for a more permanent location. The introduction of agriculture led to stability.

There is little doubt that about 10,000 years ago the human diet began what was to be a radical change. Man now relied more on plant life than ever before. He never gave up eating meat. A visit to the supermarket will tell you that. But with the advent of farming, everything changed. He was no longer a carnivore. He became an omnivore.

Many writers have recognized the development of agriculture as the most important event in the history of our culture. Settling down in one place made it necessary to have a new set of rules to be able to live with one's neighbor. Since people no longer wandered, land became an important possession. It is believed that government was the natural outgrowth of the Agricultural Revolution. Even art prospered as a result of farming. With less wasted time spent tracking his food, early man could now turn his attention to loftier pursuits.

From an economic standpoint, meat-eating today is not a very efficient process. Domesticated cattle must be fed, and much of the grain produced is for that purpose. Thus, we grow crops, but rather than eat them directly, we use them to nourish cattle, which we then eat. Thus, we are still consuming those crops, but they must first be chemically processed by these living chemical laboratories, our cattle. We have added an intermediary step to the agricultural process.

It's no secret that I love to point out to my vegetarian patients that although they eat vegetables, the vegetables themselves eat meat. Have you digested that statement? The dead "meat" in the soil, with its abundance of nitrogen, by-products of the disintegration of insects and animals and other forms of meat, are what nourish the vegetation that we eat. Everyone eats meat, directly or indirectly.

In spite of the importance of agriculture to the development of our culture, not everyone believes that it was such a good thing. Physiologist Jared Diamond, writing for *Discover* in 1987, named his article, "The Worst Mistake in the History of the Human Race." I'm still not sure whether his tongue wasn't just a little into his cheek when he wrote this, but he sure made some good points. He argued that most early farmers probably produced just one starch crop, and thus, their diets became totally unbalanced. "The farmers gained cheap calories at the cost of poor nutrition." Furthermore, since they had but one crop, if it failed, it was disastrous. He also claimed that the clumping of individuals as a result of this new lifestyle encouraged disease and epidemics.

Diamond seems to think that the African Bushmen of the Kalahari Desert in southern Africa are today better off than we are. I am reminded of the movie *The Gods Must Be Crazy*, which deals with these happy people and how their lives were almost devastated when they encountered just one tiny artifact of our modern civilization, an empty Coca-Cola bottle that fell from a small airplane.

Because the beginning of agriculture was only about 10,000 years ago, and because evolutionary processes move so slowly, it is unlikely that the man of 100,000 years ago was physically much different than you are today. He was perfectly adapted to eating meat by the time he began growing things. You're probably both structurally and physically just as he was. You're an animal whose appearance is that of a vegetarian, but through eons has adapted to eating meat. Most recently you have again discovered plant foods, but that doesn't mean you're a vegetarian.

You were never willing to let go of meat. Desmond Morris, another zoologist, took note of this in his entertaining and informative best-seller of the late sixties, *The Naked Ape.*

> *We were driven to become flesh-eaters only by environmental circumstances, and now that we have the environment under control, with elaborately cultivated crops at our disposal, we might be expected to return to our ancient primate feeding patterns. In essence, this is the vegetarian . . . creed, but it has had remarkably little success. The urge to eat meat appears to have become too deep-seated. Given the opportunity to devour flesh, we are loth to relinquish the pattern.*

According to Watson, you are thus unique in the animal world. He recognizes four eating patterns: insectivores (insect-eaters), herbivores (plant-eaters), carnivores (flesh-eaters), and omnivores (mixed diet). Many animals have undergone evolutionary changes in their diets. Some have made only a single change during their history. Others have made two changes. Man is the only animal to make three such changes.

> *The only animal ever to move from insect eating to fruit picking to meat eating to eating absolutely anything. Man.*

Of course, we men (and women) lack some of the characteristics necessary to do a really good job of digesting plant foods.

It's not surprising. We've just started to eat them. We are, so to speak, trying them out. Cows, for example, are real herbivores. They digest the cellulose that makes up the main portion of fruits and vegetables. We, on the other hand, can't digest cellulose, so it passes right through us. That is not necessarily bad. Many writers (including this one) have written books extolling the virtues of eating this fibrous material. It acts as a sweeping compound to cleanse the intestinal tract.

Here was another factor in man's dependence on meat. He had evolved sufficiently from his earliest vegetarian ancestors to the point where he could not really obtain sufficient nourishment from the plant foods available. Our African relatives did not live in lush jungles, but rather in savannas that were vast, grassy plains. The plant foods available to them were limited. Many of these plants had poisonous properties, so endowed by nature to give them protection from predators. In 1972, a Purdue University horticulturist by the name of Leopold published a paper in the prestigious journal *Science* in which he detailed all the possible plant toxins that, in his opinion, would have prevented early man from living off of plants.

In addition, of the plants that were available, few could be sufficiently digested in their raw state to achieve reasonable nutritional value. Cooking was necessary before real nutritional benefit could be derived from them. Though man has possessed fire for a very long time, it is probable that it was used principally for warmth, and it does not appear that it was used for cooking much before 50,000 years ago. By then, he was well adapted to meat-eating and truly had little need for the less-desirable plant foods.

What does the future hold? Perhaps if some random mutations occur, individuals totally adapted to eating plant foods will multiply, and it's even possible that they will not be able to tolerate meat. This fourth change would result in our again becoming an herbivorous species. Don't look for it for another 30,000 to

40,000 years, though. Even a fifth dietary change is possible. At some future date, we may be eating totally manufactured foods, nutritionally perfect for us but impossible to be categorized as either animal or vegetable. Actually I don't like to speculate about the future. I haven't the slightest idea of what science will have us eating 10 years from now, let alone far into the future.

Of course, we must ask the question of whether the meat we eat today is in any way comparable to what was eaten in prehistoric times. Of course it isn't. The wild game of ancient times was not raised on ranches with "scientific feeding" and supplements such as hormones to make its meat tender and juicy. It undoubtedly contained less fat, although the most recent trend is to produce meat with lower fat content. There is no way to return to the past, although more than one writer has advocated that we do return to a Stone Age type of diet.

One of these was the explorer Stefansson, chronicled in the next chapter, who was totally enamored with the idea of eating a Paleolithic diet. He was a practical man and a prolific writer. Let's see what he had to say about all this.

# Chapter 10

# Stefansson

I'm always researching one diet or another. More often than not, it's a diet way out of the past. I'm convinced that there is much to learn from history. Still, this obsession with the eating trends and weight-loss methods of eras long gone may be more of a hobby than a vocation.

It was a number of years ago that I was in the process of trying to find all the research material on the Pennington Diet. Although I've described this diet elsewhere, a thumbnail description of it is that it was a system of weight loss used by the medical department of a major U.S. corporation and named for the doctor who developed it. The essential element of the diet was its reliance upon large amounts of meat. I'm reasonably certain that the work of Pennington was the inspiration for the Atkins diet.

That diet had been popularized by a series of articles, the first of which appeared in *Holiday Magazine* in 1950. Others followed periodically over the years. The last of these articles was written by Earl Parker Hanson. The name caught my attention.

I can't tell you why I was familiar with his name, but I did know that he was an explorer. Why should an explorer write an article about weight loss in a popular magazine?

It didn't take too much investigation to uncover the fact that among Hanson's credits, apart from exploring, was a biography of Vilhjalmur Stefansson, another explorer and one who was much more widely known. I knew much more about Stefansson than I did about Hanson. Hanson's article gave me the stimulus to do lots of further investigation.

Anthropologists have taught us about our meat-eating origins, but it was the Arctic explorer Stefansson who probably taught us the most about how modern man handles meat-eating. Stefansson was really sort of an anthropologist. He studied the subject and was actually hired as a "cultural anthropologist" on his first Arctic expedition.

His academic life began at a prep school of the University of North Dakota in 1903, but he eventually graduated from the University of Iowa. He, like so many other young people, had a hard time deciding what direction to follow. He considered a career as a poet, worked as a reporter, went on to the divinity school at Harvard, and finally switched to archaeology there. After serving as an archeologist on an exploration to his parents' homeland, Iceland, he garnered some notice and was hired to work on a future expedition to the Arctic.

The terms of his employment called for him to meet the rest of the expedition at a specified location in the frozen wasteland of northwest Canada. The early 1900s were still dangerous times for sea travel, and as luck would have it, Stefansson, while en route to a rendezvous with the expedition, was shipwrecked and never did make contact with them. He could have sought help from the Royal Canadian Mounted Police, but instead he took the opportunity to sponge off of the Eskimos of the Mackenzie River Delta, an area of Canada's Northwest Territory, not too far east of the Point Barrow region of the northern coast of Alaska. He saw this as an opportunity to study a "primitive" people as no other scientist had ever done.

He remained a guest of the Eskimos for 18 months and completely integrated himself into their community. He learned to speak their language, hunt and fish, and was totally separated from the "civilized" world he had known.

A true scientist, Stefansson noticed everything and took voluminous and detailed notes. In his first book, *My Life with the Eskimo*, he expands on these notes to give the world its most in-depth look at the lives of what he refers to as "Stone-Age People."

It was probably this period in his life more than any other that directed his interest to how man survives under seemingly hostile conditions. Naturally, a most important element in survival is diet, so intentionally or not, he became one of the earliest nutritionists. He may not have recognized this, but it is apparent from his many books that the food of man was almost an obsession with him.

Like most people from developed countries, he had preconceived ideas of what constituted a healthful diet. He had previously written in *Harper's Magazine* of the prevailing nutritional dicta of that time:

> *To be healthy you need a varied diet, composed of elements from both the animal and vegetable kingdoms. . . . It was desirable to eat fruits and vegetables, including nuts and coarse grains. The less meat you ate the better for you.*

He must have known from the beginning that you do not have access to many fruits and vegetables in the frozen Arctic, but he also must have had a great deal of confidence in himself. After all, the people he was living with had survived without these foods, so he was determined to do the same. Since he had no idea how short or long his vacation from civilization would last, and though he was rightfully apprehensive, his writing reflects his positive attitude.

Stefansson described his breakfast while living with a family on the Mackenzie delta:

*In the morning . . . winter-caught fish, frozen so hard that they would break like glass, were brought in to lie on the floor till they began to soften a little. One of the women would pinch them now and then until, when she found her finger indented them slightly, she would begin preparations for breakfast. First she cut off the heads, and put them aside to be boiled for the children in the afternoon (Eskimos are fond of children, and heads are considered the best part of the fish). Next best are the tails, which are cut off and saved for the children also.*

He then relates how the members of the group (including himself) would each gnaw on a half-frozen fish, "about as an American does on corn." That was it. They ate raw fish and nothing else.

After breakfast, everyone would then go fishing but would return for an early lunch, which was a duplicate of breakfast. The dinner meal at about four o'clock was different. At this meal, the fish was boiled and eaten hot, but no other foods were added.

Stefansson must have been quite disciplined because he admits that prior to that time he simply hated fish. Yet he states, "About the fourth month of my first Eskimo winter I was looking forward to every meal . . . enjoying them, and feeling comfortable when they were over."

(If you are squirming at this point in your reading, try to relax. I promise you that in no place in this book will the recommended diet include frozen raw fish, or for that matter, fish heads or tails.)

Stefansson would later make other expeditions to the Arctic. He was quite in demand. Institutions such as the American Museum of Natural History were eager to sponsor him. He continued to collect data on his "Stone-Age People." In his voluminous writings about the Eskimos, he makes it clear that they thrive on fishing and hunting (caribou, seal, bear, etc.), rarely eating foods that grow from the ground. Here is his observation:

*These months on fish were the beginning of several years when I lived on an exclusive meat diet. For I count in fish when I speak of living on meat, using "meat" and "meat diet" more as a professor of anthropology than as the editor of a housekeeping magazine. The term in this article and in like scientific discussions refers to a diet from which all things of the vegetable kingdom are absent.*

*To the best of my estimate then, I have lived in the Arctic for more than five years exclusively on meat and water. (This was not, of course, one five-year stretch, but an aggregate of that much time during ten years.) One member of my expeditions, Storker Storkersen, lived on an exclusive meat diet for about the same length of time, while there are several who have lived on it from one to three years.*

Stefansson was always anxious to tell the world how healthy Eskimos really were. He wrote repeatedly of this. Dental health was a particular interest. He maintained that among Eskimos as well as other primitive societies that ate high-protein, low-carbohydrate diets, tooth decay was nonexistent. In his book, *The Fat of the Land*, he relates how he brought 100 Eskimo skulls to the American Museum of Natural History where they were examined and no sign of tooth decay discovered.

But it was not meat alone that he believed to be the essence of the diet of humans. Although he lived and did most of his work before the most important periods of archaeological discoveries described in another chapter, he had great insight into the diet of early man. He tells us:

*We should not feel discouraged, then, if in a mere five or ten thousand years of agriculture we have not as yet grown fully reconciled, biologically, to the intrusion of large quantities of sugars, starches, vegetable proteins and vegetable fats, into a regimen that has so long consisted in the main of animal proteins and animal fats.*

In case you read this quote too fast and missed it, it is the last two words that are the most remarkable. In a nutshell, Stefansson's absolute conclusion was that we needed animal fats. In fact, he believed they were vital to our survival.

Was this some casual and hurried conclusion? The result of some innate bias? Maybe he just liked fatty meat and was looking for some rationalization to make it all right. I don't think this man would do such a thing. His scientific observations of the effects of diets with varying amounts of fats on Eskimos, his own men, and himself are thorough and well documented.

He meticulously described every type of animal fat that he encountered: whale, walrus, and seal blubber; caribou fat from the animal's back, behind the eyes, and on top of the kidneys; the differences in the fat from the marrow of various bones such as the humerus or the femur; the fat found in various livers of mammals and fish. He observed that primitive people as well as modern folks have their preferences when it comes to fat, and he listed these preferences in order as though he were reciting the titles of the 10 current best-selling musical hits. His book *The Fat of the Land*, a title borrowed from the Bible, was an expansion of his earlier book *Not by Bread Alone*. Added were prefaces written by the most eminent cardiologist of the time, Dr. Paul Dudley White (he was President Eisenhower's doctor) and probably the most widely read nutritionist, Dr. Frederick J. Stare. The book was a celebration of and a monument to fat as well as to meat.

Stefansson felt that his years of experience in the Arctic supplied him with absolute proof that when men were subjected to a diet consisting of only meat, a diet devoid of carbohydrate (fruit, vegetables, and grains), it was essential that there be a sufficient amount of fat included with the meat. He even calculated that under these conditions, fat should account for 75 to 80 percent of the total calories. You might wish to contrast this with the current recommendations of the "experts" who set the percentage of calories from fat in a good diet at about 30 percent.

In his various books, Stefansson recounts multiple examples of where he, his men, or Eskimos had sufficient meat but could not obtain fat. They developed malaise, became extremely weak, and were saved only by eventually obtaining some fat or oil.

For the Eskimos of this period who relied on caribou meat, the worst time was November for the bulls or May for the cows, times when the animals were at their leanest. When eating the meat of those animals, they generally supplemented it with oil obtained from other times of the year or from other sources. The goal was always to kill the fattest animal. The Eskimos were particularly fond of the marrow on the long bones because of its good flavor and high fat content. Compare this with our love of fatty meat. Do you agree that we like fatty meat?

You may not even be aware that you like fat. The fat in our "quality" meat may be hidden from you. In general our Department of Agriculture, when it grades meat, looks at the fat content. What is called Prime, the highest grade, is the fattest, although you may not be able to visualize the fat because it is dispersed throughout the muscle. Knowledgeable steak eaters look for well "marbled" meat, though trends seem to bounce back and forth.

Today, for a nutritional adviser to suggest that you follow a diet in which 80 percent of the calories come from fat would be considered lunacy. Have things really changed that much? This bias was not that unusual 50 to 100 years ago. Certainly the human organism hasn't changed in that time. Is it possible that enormous harm was being done to those eaters of fatty meat with no clue it was happening?

Stefansson retired from exploration at age 39 and devoted the rest of his life to consulting, writing, lecturing, and tending to his library, the most complete source of information on the Arctic. He was in demand as a consultant on various matters having to do with cold climates, specifically the areas he had explored. The governments of the United States and Canada used his services. He produced an Arctic manual for the U.S. Air Force.

About 10 years after returning from his last exploration, he was the subject of one of the most interesting medical experiments ever done in the field of nutrition. Performed at New York's Bellevue Hospital, it made headlines at the time but is virtually forgotten today.

A lecture Stefansson gave to a group of doctors at the Mayo Clinic in 1920 probably led to that important study. He talked about nutrition and meat and what his diet consisted of during the time he spent in the Arctic. It aroused interest, and one of the Mayo brothers invited him to stay and be examined by the clinic. He was a curiosity. Here was a rare find: a man who had lived for years virtually exclusively on meat.

His many commitments required that he decline. I suspect that this greatly disappointed him because the prospect of convincing such a prestigious bunch of medical men that they had been wrong about their nutritional beliefs must have been enticing. A similar opportunity arose later.

In the July 3, 1926, issue of the *Journal of the American Medical Association*, Dr. Clarence W. Lieb, a well-known gastroenterologist in New York, authored a paper detailing a thorough physical examination he had given Vilhjalmur Stefansson. Stefansson's name had wide recognition; otherwise, no one would have cared whether some meat-eater were healthy or not. The article highlighted the fantastic condition he was in. It spoke of his excellent physical and mental well-being and included such particulars as his lack of constipation and the fact that his hair had thickened during his meat-eating times.

The article in *JAMA* did not escape the attention of the meat industry. According to Stefansson, the Institute of American Meat Packers asked permission to reprint the article and get it into the hands of physicians around the country. This started the wheels spinning in Stefansson's head. Here was an opportunity.

He refused their request but made them a counteroffer. He requested that they supply the funds for a real experiment to study the effects of meat-eating on humans, and they went for it.

Bellevue Hospital in New York, as one of the nation's foremost hospitals, was chosen as the site. There were to be only two subjects, Stefansson and another, younger explorer named Karsten Andersen. The idea was to study the two subjects over a one-year period during which they were to eat only meat.

The whole affair was to be supervised by a most prestigious group of scientists and physicians. Three were from Harvard, two from Johns Hopkins, and one from the American Museum of Natural History. There was a doctor from Cornell and another from the University of Chicago, as well as Lusk and DuBois, who were world famous in the field of nutrition. The meat packers also provided their own scientist, and the whole project was under the supervision of Dr. Pearl from Johns Hopkins and Dr. Lieb, the author of the *JAMA* article.

After the usual round of meetings and planning sessions, the protocol was set and Stefansson and Andersen entered Bellevue early in 1928. Aside from undergoing exhausting medical testing, for the first three weeks, they were fed a "mixed" diet with all the usual things: fruits, vegetables, cereals, meat, etc. They spent hours in glass coffin-like instruments called calorimeters, which purportedly measured their metabolism. During these three weeks, they came and went as they chose, but at the end of this preliminary period, they were put under lock and key. "Neither of us was permitted at any time, day or night, to be out of sight of a doctor or nurse."

In this phase they were actually placed on different diets. Andersen was allowed to eat any meat his heart desired. It was agreed that during that year, "meat" would include beef, pork, veal, chicken, brains, liver, and others, in short, anything that was not plant food. Eggs and milk were excluded by agreement. Stefansson, in contrast, was to eat "chopped, fatless muscle," a prospect that troubled him. He remembered times in the Arctic when he and others had become quite ill when they could not get enough fat with their meat. Nonetheless, he agreed, expecting that as before, he would begin to fare poorly in a few weeks.

He didn't have to wait that long. On the second day, he began to feel ill and reasoned that at Bellevue, they were meticulous in removing the fat, whereas during rough times in the Arctic, there was still a small amount of fat in his meat. He wrote:

> *The symptoms brought on at Bellevue by an incomplete meat diet (lean without fat) were exactly the same as in the Arctic, except that they came on faster—diarrhoea and a feeling of general baffling discomfort.*
>
> . . .
>
> *Dr. DuBois now cured me . . . by giving me fat sirloin steaks, brains fried in bacon fat, and things of that sort. In two or three days, I was all right, but I had lost considerable weight.*

His diet continued rather uneventfully for three weeks in spite of much negative comment in the press. At the onset, a well-known European nutritionist touring the United States visited them and predicted they could not last on that diet for more than four or five days. Friends of Stefansson were terribly worried that he had gone too far in donating his life to science. Yet things went well.

At the end of three weeks, he was given what he called his "parole." He had many commitments to work on other projects, to travel, and to lecture, and he was allowed to leave with the solemn promise that he would never deviate from the meat diet. There are no reports that he ever did. He was required to show up frequently for continuing tests, which he did.

Andersen remained there for 13 weeks, after which he, too, was given his parole. There was one sour note involving Andersen. There was a pneumonia epidemic at that time in New York, and the hospital was full of those patients. Before you ask, "So what?" remember that there were no antibiotics at that time. People died when they developed pneumonia. Of the pneumonia patients in the hospital, 50 percent died. Andersen survived.

On March 8, 1929, the experiment came to an end. Both men had been studied to the limit. In the July 6, 1929, issue of the *Journal of the American Medical Association*, Dr. Lieb published his summary of the findings. The paper avoided any judgments as to whether the diet was good or bad, but rather simply reported on the condition of the two subjects. The clear implication was that they came out of the test as well as or a little better than when they went in.

One little observation certainly might have aroused curiosity:

*Andersen noted that his hair stopped falling out shortly after the meat diet was started.*

The weight changes in the two men were not very remarkable. It was emphasized that during the experiment, both had led very sedentary lives. By the time it was over, Andersen had lost about four pounds and Stefansson about nine.

Of more interest was the relationship of protein to fat in their diet. They estimated that carbohydrate in the meat may have ranged from 20 to 50 grams a day, an amount that sounds high to me. Stefansson ate an average of 2,650 calories a day, 2,100 coming from fat and 550 from protein. Andersen ate 2,620 calories a day, 2,100 from fat and 510 from protein.

The bottom line: two men lived for an entire year with fat accounting for about 80 percent of their calorie intake, and they seemed to come out of it unscathed.

The cholesterol levels of both men did not change during the experiment.

Seven years later Dr. Lieb published a retrospective in the *American Journal of Digestive Diseases and Nutrition*. He reaffirmed that both men were still very healthy and showed no ill effects of their past dietary excursions.

Stefansson was always involved in some venture. A major project of his was to produce a "perfect food," something that was compact, full of nourishment, and palatable. It would have been valuable to explorers, soldiers, campers, etc.

The fact is that Stefansson didn't have to invent anything. It already existed and it was around and in use before he was born. The name of this food was pemmican. Have you ever heard of pemmican? You can't really find it today, although the name has been borrowed and is used by various products that bear no relationship to the real thing.

Pemmican was invented a long time ago by North American Indians. The product that Stefansson knew probably evolved after much trial and error. Essentially it is lean meat that is completely dried out, mixed with animal fat, and compressed into flat cakes.

Dried meat has been a staple of explorers, hunters, and other outdoor people for a long time. Jerky in the United States and Canada and biltong in South Africa are examples of dried meat. While traveling in South Africa, I had the opportunity to taste various types of biltong made from beef, veal, and antelope. I loved it. It's great exercise for your jaw muscles. By drying out or dehydrating meat, you can cut its volume down to one sixth of its original size and still maintain the same nutritional value. Pemmican, by contrast, is even more concentrated and, for its weight and volume, has more nutritional value.

Here's how, according to Stefansson, the Indians made real pemmican.

> *[T]he Indian removed every trace of fat, split the lean into thin sheets, and hung it up for wind drying. Some was dried in tepee smoke and, if there was a great hurry or if the season was wet, they parched it over a small fire.*
>
> *When thoroughly dry, the lean was converted into pounded meat, from which were removed all tendons and other bits hard to chew. Bags were made of the hide of the animal in question . . . about the size of our usual pillow cases.*
>
> *These pillow-sized rawhide bags were filled loosely with the pounded meat, as we fill pillow cases with feathers. Suet was then tried out and the rendered fat brought to nearly the temperature we use in frying doughnuts.[1] In this highly liquid state it was poured into the bag, so as to percolate everywhere.*

He goes on to tell us that the bag was sewn closed before the fat hardened; then it was pressed and pounded until it was about six inches thick. Because there was no moisture in it at all, these 90 pound bags of pemmican would keep without refrigeration for 20 years or longer.

At any time, a piece could be cut off and eaten. Each pound represented what was originally three pounds of lean meat plus one-half pound of fat. A man doing heavy labor could live well on two pounds of pemmican a day. This would be the equivalent of eating seven to eight pounds of steak.

Stefansson worked feverishly during World War II to have pemmican approved and used as a food for soldiers in the field.

---

[1] *Tried* means rendered or melted in order to obtain the oil.

After all, it was *the* food of explorers and Indians, people who were experts in survival. He stated his case eloquently in an article he published in *The Military Surgeon*. With the support of high-ranking military men, he was able to get the military to test it, and in spite of all his efforts and his considerable prestige, he was unsuccessful. Apparently, the aesthetic considerations outweighed the practical. Pemmican looks more like cow chips than it does food. Stefansson was frustrated and defeated, but he never stopped trying.

What did it taste like? Stefansson claimed it was delicious. He loved to quote Admiral Perry, who led many Arctic expeditions. He said:

> *Of all the foods I am acquainted with, pemmican is the only one that, under appropriate conditions, a man can eat twice a day for three hundred and sixty-five days in a year and have the last mouthful taste as good as the first.*[2]

> . . .

> *And it is the most satisfying food I know. . . . By the time I had finished the last morsel, I would not have walked around the completed igloo for anything or everything that the St. Regis, the Blackstone, or the Palace Hotel could have put before me.*

How is that for a testimonial? My curiosity got the best of me, and since you can't really buy pemmican, I had no choice but to attempt to make it. It was an interesting project. I did vary the formula in that I couldn't bring myself to use all that animal fat, so I substituted my own combination of vegetable oils to effect what I felt was the most desirable combination of monounsaturated and polyunsaturated fats. I compressed it into little two-inch squares about a half inch thick. They looked like brownies but tasted unmistakably like meat.

---

[2] Perry's men were given only two meals a day.

My pemmican exploit was a success. I loved it. I'm sure I am biased. I had read so much about pemmican that I expected to enjoy it. I've made it many times since, although I have to tell you, it's a real task. However, I must say that many acquaintances of mine also found it very good.

The point of dwelling on such subjects is to give you a feeling for some of the ideas from the past that would not be fashionable today. Given today's concern about cholesterol, no one would dream of telling you to concentrate meat into a compressed cake mixed with a considerable amount of fat, even if it were vegetable fat or devoid of trans fat.

Stefansson never stopped proselytizing for meat. He passed his last years as a resident expert at Dartmouth College, where his eating habits were continually under scrutiny.

He is oft alluded to and quoted. Dr. Blake Donaldson mentioned him in his diet writings. So did Dr. Pennington and many others. Even Dr. Atkins paid homage to Stefansson.

If he were alive today, I think we would all be treated to front-row seats at a real battle. I don't think he could have avoided diving into the cholesterol issue.

# Chapter 11

# Consensus through the Ages

I've always had an interest in the historical view of excess weight, particularly in how it was regarded by our ancestors. I've searched various libraries for anything that would give me a hint as not only to how excess weight was regarded at various periods in history, but more important, how it was treated. "Treated," of course, suggests some sort of intervention aimed at reversing it. Before that could happen, there had to be a reason for reversing it. Excess weight would have to have been viewed as undesirable, perhaps something to be avoided, or even something of which one should be ashamed.

The Bible offers little clues as to the prevalence, the cause, or even attitudes toward obesity. A phrase from Proverbs almost suggests that obesity is not all that bad.

*[B]ut he that putteth his trust in the Lord shall be made fat.*

I'm not a biblical scholar. I'll leave it to you to interpret that.

Obviously, standards of beauty, particularly feminine beauty, have changed over the years. Artworks, such as paintings and sculptures, certainly chronicle this change. The ancient Greeks as well as the Romans certainly focused on physical beauty for both genders. By the seventeenth century, at least European attitudes, as evidenced by the art of the time, certainly indicate a standard that our modern culture would regard as perhaps a little more than "pleasingly plump." Even the irregular dimpling of fatty tissue that has now come to be known as "cellulite" was evident in many paintings that proclaimed feminine beauty. I can't recall any paintings or sculptures prior to the nineteenth century displaying any form resembling a supermodel.

The paintings of such artists as Peter Paul Rubens, who produced his enormous canvases well into the seventeenth century, must have been representative of what his admirers also admired. Rubens seemed to like his female subjects to be "full-figured."

There are some interesting milestones relating to the weight of humans that we just take for granted. When you step on the scale and look down (or, in my office, up) at those numbers and either smile or frown depending on what you see, you might take it for granted that that is how it's always been. True, we were weighing things way back in biblical times, but we were not weighing people. It wasn't until about 1600, when a doctor from Padua, Italy, Santorio Santorio, actually weighed a human and assigned a number to the result. I believe he himself was the first *weighee*. Santorio S. was a pretty smart fellow. He was studying the relationship between the weights of the things we eat and drink and also expel (that is, feces and urine), and how they relate to our own weights. He's sometimes credited with being the father of the study of metabolism.

Getting into the twentieth century, there was a definite shift. I'm sure you've seen photos or drawings of the flat-chested flapper of the 1920s. She was perhaps even skinnier than today's fashion models. That era was just a little before my time . . . just a little.

Yet even back then, when a little bulk was considered desirable for ladies, the world was already looking for ways to reduce the bulk. It was only natural that doctors became involved. And with doctors' influence, the inevitable happened—diet books.

My interest in this subject naturally led me to diet books throughout the ages. I have quite a collection, hundreds, in fact. I'm not exactly sure how many. If I were to succumb to the temptation to sit down and read them for pleasure, I never would get any work done. I never would have written this book. They're fascinating as well as thought provoking, funny, stupid, unbelievable, and a few more adjectives that I don't have on the tip of my tongue.

I've searched for the very first diet book ever published. That's not easy to find. There isn't a clear-cut distinction between a book that gives menu suggestions and one devoted entirely to the subject of diet. Ancient medical writers such as Hippocrates and Galen touched on the subject, but they didn't produce a diet book.

In my opinion, the first real diet book was written in 1727, about 50 years before the American Revolution. Thomas Short, an English physician, wrote *A Discourse Concerning the Causes and Effects of Corpulency*. I actually have a copy. It's not easy to read if you're not a professor of antiquated English literature because in the type style of the day, the letter *s* looks a lot like the letter *f*. Once you get past that hurdle, it's really quite humorous.

He certainly doesn't confine his advice to diet alone. In one early passage, he explains how healthy human beings come to be born. It starts with their parents:

> *I shall lay down some signs of a healthy State and long Life: But to come to the Knowledge of these, we must gather our Observations as far back as the Womb; nay, as the Act of Coitus, wherein we were begotten.*
>
> *1. Persons must be generated of healthy, vigorous parents, that are come to full Age, who have rarely used Venery; but*

*when they set to it, did it with Heat, Strength, full Desire,
and in the Morning, after sound Sleep, perfect Digestion,
especially in the Spring of the Year.[1]*

I wonder if he was planning a marriage manual in the future.

Just as I'm shocked seeing how obesity is increasing with every
passing year, it seems that Short shared the same concern:

*[N]o Age did ever afford more instance of Corpulency than
our own . . .*

If I were to attempt to summarize Short's approach to weight
loss, I'm afraid I'd fail. It was so vague and disjointed as to qualify
as no advice at all. The reader was advised to eat "Bread of Oats,
Rye, or Barley" with no particular quantity specified. For beverages,
"mild and smooth" liquors, and certainly "Stale Ale or Beer" that
he maintains

*. . . quietly stimulates the Fibres, invigorates the Solids,
promotes Digestion and Perspiration; and by use of this
Method I have known some lose two Stone of fat [that's
28 pounds] in one Week's Time.*

I don't know how you feel about it, but I don't want my "fibres"
stimulated or my solids invigorated. As for losing 28 pounds in a
week—not if I have to drink stale beer to do it.

This guy was a respected member of the Royal Society of
Physicians. This was professional advice. Can you imagine what
the quacks were recommending? He did proffer one weight-loss
tip that quite a few people follow today but not always to their
advantage. He did advise, "Smoking of Tobacco."

A few years later in 1757, Dutch physician Malcolm Flemyng
presented his paper, "A Discourse on the Nature, Causes, and Cures

---

[1] To paraphrase Woody Allen: Venery is only dirty when it's done right.

of Corpulency," before the Royal Society of Physicians in London. He was one of the first to suggest a genetic, although he certainly didn't use the term, connection to one's obesity. He felt that some people were more apt to be fat than others. As for the "Cures" part, can't you guess? Soap. It washes all that fat out of your body. He had keenly observed that soap did that to his linens. It's not much of a step to apply that to humans. Flemyng said eat (or drink) soap. I confess, I haven't tried it, and please don't you.

Then came a German who said the only things that can be used by the body for energy are carbohydrates and fats. What about protein? It was used to construct the body or to repair it but not to run it. That's not a silly observation. It's rather clever. You can see how he got that idea. After all, we are essentially built of protein. He must have known that the carbohydrate and fat get "burned up." They are our fuel (our energy). The idea was very smart but wrong. Nonetheless, he could actually have been the father of the high-protein diet. (A later fellow, Banting, whom you will soon hear more about, usually gets the credit.) Quite a few years later, in the nineteenth century, a very famous scientist of the time, Claude Bernard, told us that protein could also serve as a source of energy.

William Wadd was an early nineteenth-century surgeon who had a multifaceted career. He had enough prestige to be appointed as one of the personal surgeons to George IV. He issued his *Cursory Remarks on Corpulence* in 1810, and they were indeed cursory since they gave no more advice on how to beat hunger when on a low-calorie diet than do the diet books of today. Essentially, he moralized. He regarded abstinence from food as a virtuous goal and the giving in to hunger as a sign of moral weakness. Wadd promulgated just another example of the kind of advice that could work but in the real world doesn't because people, by their nature, won't follow it.

To Wadd's credit, he did renounce Flemyng's use of soap as a reducing agent. He said that salt did a better job!

In 1834, Sylvester Graham, an ordained minister from Maine, embarked on a series of lectures recommending to the world the eating of a healthful diet. For some reason he was quite controversial, and his lectures occasionally ended in near riots. Could it be that the public objects to being told to eat a *healthful* diet? I don't think that he did much for the science of the treatment of obesity, but he did have one great accomplishment. Have you ever wondered how graham crackers got their name? Now you know.

It's generally believed that high-protein diets result in faster weight loss, and as a group, over the past 140 or so years, they have probably been the most widely used of all the reducing diets.

The first of these to have achieved real notoriety was the Banting Diet, which probably should have been named the Harvey Diet, for it was Dr. William Harvey, a London ear specialist, who invented it. Banting, it turns out, was his patient.

William Banting was a not-so-humble coffin maker whose handiwork had served as permanent enclosures for some of England's most illustrious. In 1862 he published his book, actually not much more than a pamphlet, describing the method by which he had lost weight. His *Letter on Corpulence, Addressed to the Public* has become somewhat of a classic, if not an oddity, among medically related books. It was perhaps an early example of a "how-to" book written for the public to help solve some medical problem.

Banting's greatest problem was his weight, which he quite vociferously denounced as a great inconvenience. His book begins as follows:

> *Of all the parasites that affect humanity I do not know of, nor can I imagine, any more distressing than that of Obesity . . .*

That pretty well set the tone of the book. His purpose in writing it was to tell the world how he had successfully lost his corpulence by following the dietary advice of his wonderful doctor, and then altruistically donating this information to the masses. Mysteriously, he did not name the doctor in the first edition of his book although he did promise to supply the name to anyone in earnest who wrote to him.

Dr. Harvey had been consulted originally not because of Banting's weight problem, but rather because of a hearing loss. It was actually Banting's second try at getting help with his hearing, having dismissed an earlier ear doctor whom he felt was not thorough enough. He discovered that Dr. Harvey was indeed the right man.

> *I found the right man, who unhesitatingly said he believed my ailments were caused principally by corpulence, and prescribed a certain diet . . .*

This was not Banting's first try at losing weight either. He had tried a variety of cures other than diet. Neither Turkish baths nor exercise worked for him. He complained that previous dietary instructions had been too general. "Moderation and light food" had been advised. Dr. Harvey's very specific instructions were obviously preferable.

When Banting first consulted Harvey, he was 202 pounds, 5 feet 5 inches tall, and 66 years of age. He states that he lost about a pound a week and at the time of writing his book was down to 167 pounds. He expresses his assurance that in "a few more weeks [I] will fully accomplish the object for which I have laboured." He was, of course, delighted with the weight loss, and he mentioned almost as an afterthought that there was also "immense effect and advantage . . . to my hearing . . ."

The diet that Banting followed was probably the first published high-protein diet. You'll be disappointed with its details.

He was told to abstain from bread, butter, milk, sugar, beer, and potatoes. Here, in his own words, is what he was instructed to eat:

*For breakfast, I take four or five ounces of beef, mutton, kidneys, broiled fish, bacon, or cold meat of any kind except pork; a large cup of tea (without milk or sugar), a little biscuit, or one ounce of dry toast.*

*For dinner, Five or six ounces of any fish except salmon, any meat except pork, any vegetable except potato, one ounce of dry toast, fruit out of a pudding, any kind of poultry or game, and two or three glasses of good claret, sherry, or Madeira—Champagne, Port and Beer forbidden.*

*For supper, Three or four ounces of meat or fish, similar to dinner, with a glass or two of claret.*

*For nightcap, if required, A tumbler of grog—(gin, whisky, or brandy, without sugar)—or a glass or two of claret or sherry.*

This was obviously a meat diet or more correctly a meat and alcohol diet. You have to wonder if Banting didn't modify Harvey's instructions just a little bit. But this is the diet that he says he followed, and there seems to be little reason to doubt the success that he claimed.

Interestingly enough, he includes a familiar admonition, one found in most diet books:

*I do not recommend every corpulent man to rush headlong into such a change of diet, (certainly not), but act advisedly and after full consultation with a physician.*

I can't argue with that advice, and as you will see, I dwell upon that subject, returning repeatedly to it in the course of this book.

Banting obviously liked the diet because it told him exactly what to do. As I look at it, it is not all that specific. I would have preferred that he had let me know how "little" was his little biscuit, how much of the vegetables was prescribed, and what is "fruit out of a pudding." Even what seems specific is not. After enunciating the diet, he states that he is not "strictly limited to any quantity at either meal." He's clear enough about the beverages, however. They might have been Banting's favorite part of the diet.

No one can question Banting's sincerity and his gratitude to Dr. Harvey. He unselfishly supplied the first edition of his book free and sold later editions at his own cost.

This simple book and these uncomplicated instructions were the backbone of reducing diets for at least the next 100 years. "Bantingism" was debated in academic circles but was for the most part accepted as the standard method of weight reducing among the common people. It was not that everyone adhered to Banting's exact instructions, but a high-protein, low-carbohydrate diet with very limited fat was obviously the method of choice.

*The Lancet* was and still is England's stodgy but excellent general weekly medical journal. It has been around longer than even your great-grandfather can remember. *The Lancet* did its share of editorializing on Bantingism. About a year after Banting first published, unsigned articles began appearing, castigating Banting and his diet. The article in the May 7, 1964, issue, after tearing him apart bit by bit, closed with the following:

> *We advise Mr. Banting, and everyone of his kind, not to meddle with medical literature again, but be content to mind his own business.*

I think there is great significance in one of the sentences in the article, for it reflects an attitude that may be as fresh as if it had been uttered yesterday.

> *But if every person who so obtains relief were immediately to publish a pamphlet about his ailment, and about the doctor who cured him, it would inflict grave mischief on the profession, lowering its dignity, and giving rise to unworthy suspicions.*

In spite of this harsh criticism, that sentence does seem to admit to the fact that Banting did get "relief." Are they admitting that the diet was successful?

About five months later, another editorial in the same journal took a more moderate approach. It disapproved of the diet because not enough research had been done on it, and it advocated further investigation. Four weeks later, in the October 29th issue, another editorial acknowledged that the use of the diet was widespread. It seemed to be straining to find objections to Bantingism. It declared that Banting's diet didn't contain enough fat, a deficiency that "impairs the nutrition of the nervous system."

In the years that followed, textbooks generally alluded to the Banting Diet. It was often suggested as one of the alternative weight-loss programs. In some books, it was criticized.

Did Banting's diet challenge the general theory dealing with calories and weight? It's hard to say. The diet was so indefinite that we can't assign a calorie count to it.

What, then, was so revolutionary about this diet? Why did it receive so much attention? If it were published today, it wouldn't even be noticed. That's because every month 100 new diets make it into the magazines, into the bookstores, and on to the Internet. We have come to expect a new diet every time we turn around. We've become jaded with the avalanche of diets.

To understand what was so revolutionary, you must understand how primitive was the dietary advice of that period. What made Banting's pamphlet so extraordinary is that it actually told the reader what to eat in rather definite terms. That was revolutionary. What Banting really said was that all you have to do to lose weight is eat this and this and this. Furthermore, there were other things you shouldn't eat. You shouldn't eat this and this. That was different. And the public loved it.

There is no question that Banting's (or Harvey's) high-protein diet also set the tone for the diets of the first half of the twentieth century. High protein was in. A popular notion mentioned in many of the medical texts was the concept of the specific dynamic action of protein. It was believed, correctly, that we use some calories in the process of digesting our food but very few in the case of fats and carbohydrates. Protein was a different story. Protein used more calories in the digestive process than it supplied. Thus, by eating pure protein, you would create a calorie deficit and lose weight. The concept was discredited and died somewhere down the line. I'm not all that sure that there wasn't some truth in it. It would certainly help to explain why some people have lost weight over the years.

On October 6, 1888, a letter written by Dr. W. Towers-Smith, was printed in the *British Medical Journal*. The *BMJ* printed lots of letters from doctors. Through journals, doctors communicated their success and failures to their colleagues. Remember, this was before radio, television, or even telephones. The Internet? Forget it. To communicate, you had to appear in print.

The interchange of letters in journals over the years could be described as nothing less than cute. The British have always had this delightful way of making disapproval sound like approval, so as an American, you have to read carefully. These letters, back and forth, can amuse me for hours.

Towers-Smith, in his letter, relates the diet that he put himself on three years previous:

> *On March 1, 1885, I weighed, in the Jermyn Street Turkish Bath, 15 stones 10 pounds: on the 2nd I commenced the treatment, which was as follows:—Breakfast: one pound rump steak, without fat. Lunch: another pound of rump steak. At dinner: one pound of grilled cod and one pound of rump steak. I drank at intervals during the twenty-four hours a gallon of hot water.*

About two weeks into the diet, he admits that he reduced the quantity of meat and added some toast but changed nothing else but beverages. In one month he was down to 179 pounds. Remember that a stone is 14 pounds, so his original weight was 220 pounds. Thus, he went from 220 pounds down to 179 in 30 days. Dropping 41 pounds in one month is dramatic in anyone's book. He then tells how he had since put 40 patients on the diet "with equal success." The rest of the letter went on to say how great he and his patients felt.

This apparently opened the floodgates. Going through future issues of the *BMJ*, I counted between that time and February 6, 1892, 10 more letters from Towers-Smith and 11 from others responding to him. (With no TV to entertain them, the readers must have viewed this exchange as we do a soap opera.)

On November 10, 1888, Towers-Smith went into detail on his 40 patients, and the table of results was indeed impressive. He indicated that only one person out of the bunch dropped out, refusing to conform to the diet.

Most of the letters responded approvingly, but there were a few negative responses from doctors who felt the diet was too narrow for patient acceptance. Towers-Smith obviously disagreed and published further good results of his treatment.

Could such a bizarre regimen produce the results reported? Careful reading of all the letters convinced me that Towers-Smith could not have gotten away with deceptive reporting over such a long period of time in the *BMJ*. I believe they would be wary of publishing material that served as a veiled advertisement. That journal together with *The Lancet* shared an untarnished reputation in the medical community, and they command the same respect today.

Then there was the Salisbury System.

In a word, lots of weight was lost on a diet consisting of not much more than a quantity of meat, and there is no suggestion of any untoward effects.

It is a fact of history that meat diets have always been the subject of much criticism by the "authorities," yet they have always seemed to receive the approval of the masses. Perhaps that is because we humans quite simply like meat. As well as I can determine, the Salisbury System seemed to have the approval of everyone. Evidence of this approbation perhaps is its very designation as a system rather than just simply a diet. It was not a weight-loss diet as such, but rather a general curative as well as lifelong diet for everyone. Medical men of stature had no reservations in recommending this diet. Dr. J. H. Salisbury of New York, in his 1888 book, *The Relation of Alimentation and Disease,* pretty well says that his system will cure everything.

The medical literature for years to follow makes reference to the Salisbury System as one of the mainstays of the doctor's therapeutic bag of tricks. For example, Dr. E. C. Atkins (not the Atkins you have known), writing in an 1893 *Journal of the American Medical Association,* discusses the treatment of unresponsive consumption (tuberculosis):

> *But it is in this class of otherwise hopeless cases that the Salisbury beef diet proves to be of the greatest service. . . . Under its influence, the appetite becomes enormous; the patient who sickened at the sight of meat, now eats three or four pounds a day.*

Salisbury, judging from his book, was an intense fellow, perhaps even obsessive-compulsive. After reading only a few pages, it would be impossible to doubt his sincerity. He truly believed that all problems of the human race were caused by what we eat. He did meticulous research to prove his point. In his words, here was the beginning of a whole series of experiments:

> *In September, 1856, I engaged six strong, healthy men, in the vigor of life, ranging in age from 25 to 40 years, to feed upon a special line of diet solely, with the understanding that I would pay them $30 per month each, if they submitted faithfully to the rigid discipline laid down.*

At that time, $30 was easily a living wage because it included room and board. You see, Salisbury had enticed these men to live in his home so he could study them in great detail. Meals were included, but therein lay the catch to his scheme. Aside from the fact that the living arrangement today would be regarded with suspicion, it is possible that conditions in the house during the initial diet phase were less than ideal since the diet consisted of only one food: baked beans.

Salisbury's plan was to feed his guests one food at a time for various periods and to study them intensely, recording every aspect of their physical condition, even to the extent of collecting and analyzing each bowel movement. The pages of organized charts of the detailed description of the latter are a marvel of personal dedication.

From baked beans, he went on to oats, then to a sequence of one food after another but always only one at a time. Of course, he did not keep the original crew of paid guests. They were constantly replaced with others as they dropped out. They were always men. I suppose that to house women during that period of our history would have been unseemly behavior.

From this came the ideal diet for sick humans, a diet that was liberalized and modified for the well individual. It takes only four words to describe it: hot water and beef.

Salisbury had a formidable following. His regimen seemed to work. Believers came from far and wide. The famous socialist, novelist, playwright, and general reformer Upton Sinclair, in his biography, tells how after a lifetime of "stomach trouble" and having tried every nutritional gimmick that existed, including vegetarianism, in 1909 he switched to the Salisbury System.

Salisbury's fame crossed the ocean and an erudite English lady, Elma Stuart, claiming that she owed her life to him and his system, wrote a book entitled *What Must I Do to Get Well? and How Can I Keep So?* It was subtitled, *An Exposition of the Salisbury Treatment,*

and it certainly was that. Her book went through umpteen printings. She actually outdid Salisbury in thoroughness. Her book was
charming and a joy to read, but then again, I've always been a
sucker for 1889 books.

She recognizes three states of health: the Sick, the Seedy, and
the Well. I knew you were going to ask me about that, so I will tell
you what my dictionary says about *seedy*. It means "physically run
down" or "under the weather." Once I had looked it up, I realized
that the term had been familiar to me after all.

Here's the diet. For the sick, take four pints of hot water spaced
throughout the day. The solid part of the diet, according to Elma,
is as follows:

> *The meat for this purpose . . . from the round or flank . . .*
> *freshly killed. . . . The plan is to have the raw beef finely*
> *minced by sending it through a machine three times. All fat,*
> *gristle, connective tissue to be completely scraped away . . . the*
> *mince to be made up very sloppily into cakes; seasoned with*
> *black pepper and salt . . . moistened with good soup . . .*

She goes on to explain that they must be "grilled well through,
lightly on both sides, over a clear fire. How much does one eat of
this? As much as one wants but "always leaving off feeling you
could eat just a little more."

As the patient's condition progresses through the seedy and
well phases, the diet is modified first by eliminating the mincing
or grinding of the beef, and by gradually adding some other foods.
Beef, however, always remains the cornerstone of the diet.

She does not dwell on weight problems but does address it
succinctly:

> *Obesity is a disease produced by over-feeding on the foods*
> *that make fat or adipose tissue. The cure is safe and simple.*
> *Stop those foods that make fat, and rigidly adhere, till the*

*disease is cured, to lean meats, broiled or roasted,—beef, mutton, lamb, game, etc. (no hardship!)*

The ending parenthetical expression is hers, not mine.

At least someone in England must have been impressed with Salisbury's diet. An 1893 item in *The Lancet* written by a physician describes his success with the diet but makes no mention of its origins or of Salisbury. I suspect that even 100 years after the liberation of "the colonies," it was still hard for some to accept that anything good could have come out of them.

When I read about dietary advice such as that of Ms. Stuart speaking for Salisbury, I cannot help but try to place myself back in that period, more than 100 years ago. Lacking our sophisticated therapies, illness of any kind must have been a frightening experience. It is easy to see how the sick would grasp for anything that would offer them hope. An extreme diet of this type is truly not that difficult to try. But the Salisbury System would have died on its own if those who followed it hadn't seen some benefit. This diet was in wide use until long after Salisbury died in 1905. Allbutt and Rolleston's *A System of Medicine*, a standard internal medicine text published in 1910, recommends the Salisbury System, advocating up to three pounds of meat a day with "no bread or vegetable food" allowed. I cannot help but think that for a therapy to persist for more than 50 years on at least two continents, there must have been some merit.

The first half of the twentieth-century evidenced a flurry of diets and other weight-loss techniques. A multitude of frauds promised miraculous transformations. There were drugs that worked but whose safety was debated. Amphetamines were controlling hunger. A chemical named dinitophenol seemed too good to be true. It raised body temperature and, thus, resulted in increased expenditure of calories, enough to overcome even overeating. It *was* too good to be true. Blindness and death turned out to be less desirable than being fat, so its use was abandoned.

Now we come to my favorite—Horace Fletcher. It's not that Fletcher ever did much for science, though he did write several books, all of which I have (and I can tell you they have provided me with hours of merriment). By the early twentieth century, everyone knew about Fletcher. They also knew about the philosophy of "Fletcherism" as well as the method of eating known as "Fletcherizing." If you're not familiar with any of this, you're in for a treat. You might even decide to Fletcherize your own food. If you do, please don't write me to tell me about it.

I'll start with a hint. He was also known as "The Great Masticator." I won't keep you waiting any longer. Fletcher believed that the way to health was to put any food that you desire in your mouth in any quantity; just don't swallow it.

Should I pause for a moment to let you, umm, *digest* that?

You certainly deserve more of an explanation than that. So you can chew to your heart's content. And you really are allowed to swallow, but you may not swallow anything that is *solid*. That leaves liquids and those food juices that trickle down your throat. Yes, now you've got it. Chew your food until it's actually a liquid; then swallow the liquid.

Of course, the longer you chew, the more liquid the stuff becomes. You must still differentiate between liquid and solid. Semiliquids don't qualify as liquids. Since we all swallow quite reflexively without any awareness of doing so, Fletcherism takes a good deal of concentration, but Fletcher himself assures us that with a little bit of practice, you can master it.

At least one writer has suggested that Fletcher actually got the idea for Fletcherism from British Prime Minister William Gladstone, who once remarked that we should chew each mouthful 32 times, once for each tooth. Fletcher obviously felt he could improve on that.

I'm sure you've already asked the obvious question. What do you do with the stuff that you are not permitted to swallow?

Well, first of all, you are ordered to do a lot of chewing, a task that makes any meal consequently quite long. He recommends about 100 chews per minute. That's more than one a second. You're not to stop chewing until you are sure that further mastication of the food will produce no further changes in it.

Oh, yes, what do you then do with it? Well, what would you expect to do with it? You spit it out, dummy.

There you have Fletcherism in a nutshell. Chew, chew, chew, then spit.

Fletcher himself is said to have Fletcherized his food fanatically for most of his life. And what did he have to show for it?

Let's get into who Fletcher was. First of all, he was American importer, and as a food lecturer, he became a millionaire. He eventually left his humble surroundings to live in a palace in Venice. Fletcherism was certainly good to him.

In his writing he tells us that Fletcherizing food was also good for his health. Before he began Fletcherizing, he weighed 200 pounds and was turned down for life insurance. Afterward, and rather quickly, he got down to 165 and became well insured.

Above all, he was a promoter. He promoted himself, mainly, along with Fletcherism. He loved to boast about how strong he had become by chewing and spitting. At age 56, he went off to the Yale University gymnasium, where, under experimenter's supervision, he competed for strength and endurance against Yale's best athletes. Guess who won?

The names of those who Fletcherized are legend: John D. Rockefeller, Upton Sinclair, Mark Twain, Henry James, and lots of lesser-known folk.

Indeed, Fletcher made himself a celebrity. Don't celebrities get frequent invitations to dinner parties? Would you want a spitter at your dinner table? I'm not too sure where he did his spitting. Maybe with a little more research, I'll find out and cover that in my next book.

He was equally intense about examining his stools. I get the sense that he was never quite satisfied with them, even though he boasted about their charm and how free they were of unpleasant odor. Yet he never was able to achieve absolute perfection. After all, he obviously reasoned, if you never swallow insoluble material, you should never expect to have a bowel movement. In his case, that could not have been true. What would he have had to examine?

In his 1906 book, *The New Glutton or Epicure*, he devotes a whole chapter to feces. I was particularly impressed with his willingness to tell a story that came from an unnamed physician. Apparently this medical man found himself housed with another gentleman, a prolific writer. The entire story relates to the writer's bowel functions. What follows is a small excerpt of what was said. I really did want you to read this entire book, but if you choose to skip this excerpt, I'll understand.

> *There had, under the regime above mentioned, been no evacuation of the bowels for eight days. At the end of the period he informed me that there were indications that the rectum was about to evacuate, though the material he was sure could not be of a large amount. Squatting upon the floor of the room, without any perceptible effort he passed into the hollow of his hand the contents of the rectum. This was done to demonstrate human normal cleanliness and inoffensiveness; neither stain nor odour remaining, neither in the rectum or upon the hand. The excreta were in the form of nearly round balls, varying in size from a small marble to a large plum. These were greenish-brown in colour, of firm consistence, and covered over with a thin layer of mucous; but there was no more odour to it than there is to a hot biscuit.*

Obviously Fletcher felt he could impress us with this one benefit of his diet. I was not impressed, and I have not had a hot biscuit since I read the above.

So much for Fletcher, and if you've been able to hold down your last meal, let's move on to other diets. Fletcherism was a hard act to follow, so quite a few years passed without much to write about.

In June 1949, a paper was published in the journal *Industrial Medicine.* The author, A. W. Pennington, MD, was with the medical division of the E. I. DuPont de Nemours and Company, the giant chemical manufacturer. Dr. Pennington told us that obesity costs industry money for various reasons. It predisposes its victims to a number of ailments, causing factories to lose good employees; it impairs workers' efficiency; and the low-calorie diets that are followed leave workers weak and unproductive. He went through a rather incomprehensible theory to explain obesity, then reported on 20 individuals who had lost weight on a particular diet that he had prescribed.

It was a strange paper, particularly since he gave no basis for his beliefs. He did include a table listing his 20 subjects that showed their beginning weights, their final weights, and the corresponding dates. The average weight loss was 22 pounds, but it ranged from nine pounds to 54 pounds. It took them from one to six months to lose the weight.

None of this is too startling or exciting. I generally expect my own patients to lose faster. What was startling was that he said he allowed his patients who were dissatisfied with the basic diet of 3,000 calories a day to eat unlimited extra amounts of a mixture of protein and fat. That's enough to make anyone sit up and take notice. Forgetting about the extras, how can anyone lose weight on 3,000 calories a day? Furthermore, he assured us that these people all felt great.

I really don't know how his paper was received. I suspect, not very well. I know how I would have regarded it. Because it was so sketchy and did not follow any of the rules that scientific papers are supposed to follow, I would probably have concluded that it was plain nonsense. Essentially, I would have written off Pennington as a liar and forgotten about him.

To his credit, he did get himself published in a recognized journal, and he was with the medical department of a major corporation. Presumably his 20 subjects were DuPont employees, although he didn't say so in the paper. If he were lying about the results, how could he have gotten away with it? Others in the factory would have known he was lying. You already know that I am a skeptic and perhaps a cynic, yet after reading everything Pennington wrote and evaluating his position at DuPont, I must conclude that he was telling the truth.

Here is the diet in his words:

> *The daily diet included two to three ounces of fat at each of the three meals of the day. Protein and carbohydrate, combined, were given in a minimum of three times this amount. The high protein, low carbohydrate principle was maintained.*

Fat? Can you lose weight by eating fat? Here is more of what he had to say:

> *Those who followed the diet reported increased energy and sense of well-being. Notable was the lack of hunger between meals. Objective signs of improved health were evident, particularly a reduction in blood pressure in hypertensives. Some urine tests for ketones were run, but none was found . . .*

I have not come across any immediate response, positive or negative, to Pennington's paper. Perhaps it was ignored as the ravings of some nut.

We heard about Dr. Pennington again about a year later, but this time in *Holiday* magazine. As I recall, *Holiday* was then directed to upscale folks who liked to take nice vacations. Its readers were probably the same group who wanted to be fashionably thin. *Holiday* was a high-quality magazine dealing mainly with travel. It was not the place to find either controversy or diets. A long article titled "Eat Well and Lose Weight" devoted itself to a diet designed by Dr. Pennington. In a rather light journalistic style, Elizabeth Woody, the author, opens by describing her lunch with Dr. Pennington in a hotel dining room. The two of them ate rare steak, and he encouraged her to have more if she were not satisfied. They were both allowed the French fries that accompanied it, but he added, "Don't ask for seconds."

He told her that his diet consisted of one-half pound or more of fresh meat with the fat, eaten three times a day. "The main stipulation," according to him, "is don't skip the fat. One part of fat by weight to three parts of lean, always and invariably." When the reporter reached for the salt, he stopped her.

She then described how they walked a short distance to one of the DuPont buildings, where she was introduced to Dr. George Gehrmann, head of the company's medical division. Dr. Gehrmann confirmed that this was the program followed by DuPont employees. He spoke in glowing terms of the success of the program. Dr. Pennington was described as an internist and an expert in industrial medicine. He had approached the obesity problem just as other industrial problems were tackled, and the solution worked. The 20 weight-loss subjects who had been written about a year before were part of a pilot project that was deemed a complete success. The full program was in place, and it, too, was a great triumph.

Clearly, *Holiday* magazine was advocating this reducing diet. They did more than that. They offered a 20 page booklet that they published with complete instructions on the diet for just 10 cents. Remember, that was 1949.

The Holiday Diet became famous. Some preferred to call it the Pennington Diet. Back at the factory, they probably called it the

DuPont Diet. No matter what they named it, there was no question that Pennington had rocked the boat.

Pennington wrote a number of papers after that. They were published in such journals as the *American Journal of Digestive Diseases* and *The American Journal of Clinical Nutrition*. His June 1953 lead article in the *New England Journal of Medicine*, which was actually material presented at a symposium on obesity partially sponsored by the Harvard School of Public Health, was evidence that he had indeed arrived.

In that paper, he reiterated his diet. He still maintained that one could lose weight on a meat and fat diet, with 80 percent of the calories coming from fat. His writing had become more scholarly, and he provided a number of references for his diet. I must confess that the theoretical basis for his diet was still quite a mystery to me, even though he went to lengths to explain it. I don't think it would be productive for me to try to explain the theory to you since I really don't understand it myself.

Of interest is that he mentions Dr. Blake Donaldson, of whom I shall soon speak. He also refers liberally to the Arctic explorer Stefansson who spent a sizable portion of his life eating only meat.

I don't think I can dismiss Pennington's results as easily as I can his theories. It is quite conceivable that he was doing the right things for the wrong reasons. I was in college then. I wasn't the least bit overweight, and I did not yet have an intense interest in medicine, so I did not follow these events. The name Pennington was unfamiliar to me. But members of my family and my friends were always dieting. I clearly remember that lots of people were on the Holiday Diet. I didn't even know what kind of diet it was. What I do remember is that I saw the results firsthand; people were losing weight.

Was Pennington really on to something? Or was he a nut, an opportunist, a charlatan? I don't think he could have gotten away with such a deception for a number of years while associated with DuPont. Is it possible that the employees were deceived into believing that their steaks and roast beef were causing them to lose weight? I don't think that we can question that his subjects lost weight. I think we can only conclude that they lost this weight on a number of calories that should *not* have resulted in weight loss. Yet in spite of the attention generated by Pennington, I can find but a smattering of significant research that emerged from his work.

There is no question that the medical establishment would have frowned on the commercialization of his diet by *Holiday.* Doctors, particularly in 1949, were supposed to transfer their advice to patients in their own offices, not in popular magazines. Was Pennington ignored because he openly cooperated with the *Holiday* writer? Who's to say?

If we assume that Pennington's patients lost what he said they lost, there is still the question of whether it was safe to follow that diet. We start teaching in the lower grades that fat is a no-no. The most educated advice today is to limit your fats so your waistline and your cholesterol stay in check. Even if we determine that his diet was unsafe, we should not close the door to examining the ramifications of what he observed. We should not ignore the fact that he disputes (and seems to disprove) what is generally believed about calories and the idea that calories are all that count. (See Chapter 12.) Someone should have been interested in learning why Pennington's patients supposedly lost weight on 3,000 calories a day.

There is a postscript to the Pennington story. Holiday magazine published a second article on the diet in February of 1951. It essentially dealt with the multitude of letters the magazine had received, testimonials to the success of the diet. Woody wrote:

> *I can't remember a single letter which reported getting no results when the diet was carried out conscientiously, but I do remember several that said, "I haven't been able to follow the plan exactly because . . .*

The author of the two articles closes by admitting that *she* lost 30 pounds on the diet.

Pennington had his critics within the medical establishment. Accompanying his 1951 paper in the *Delaware State Medical Journal* titled "The Use of Fat in a Weight Reducing Diet" was sort of a rebuttal by two other Wilmington, Delaware, physicians. They were polite and respectful. His work was called "very interesting." But Pennington's paper was dismissed with a restatement of the type of dogma that persists to this day:

> *Despite what Dr. Pennington says about calories, the simple principle—that obesity is invariably the result of a disproportion between the inflow and outflow of energy—remains unchallenged. Persons who ingest fewer calories than they produce lose weight. The human body does not violate the law of conservation of energy.*

They might as well have said, "Dr. Pennington is a liar." The axiom quoted was hardly unchallenged. Pennington contested it, and there was no satisfactory rebuttal. The critic refused to accept any proof that the concept of calories controlling our weights may be flawed. He stubbornly adhered to the accepted calorie manifesto and doggedly maintained that the "principle" he believed in must be accepted as part of the ground rules, and only theories that are consistent with the old rules would be heard. I'm afraid that little has changed in the 58 years that have intervened. You might expect to hear more of the same type of criticism when this book is reviewed.

The real reason for dismissing Pennington's findings can perhaps be gleaned from the discourse of his second critic in that journal:

> *I would like to say one more word, and I have previously mentioned this to Dr. Pennington, that even if we would assume that this is a good diet, and it may turn out to be*

*such, I would like to say that I was most disappointed and shocked to see the display given his diet in* Holiday *magazine, representing the work of one of the most outstanding industrial medical departments in the country. I have always been very happy associated with the individuals in the medical department of the DuPont Company, and I hope I still will. But I cannot conceive of any reason why such an organization would allow a splurge like what was displayed in* Holiday *magazine, and I certainly am sorry that it occurred.*

I can think of a reason DuPont might have allowed it; it was an accurate description of the benefits their employees had received. The "splurge" of which he speaks was a straightforward, dignified, non-flamboyant article that simply told the story.

Note also that what the gentleman seems to be saying is, even if we would assume that this is a good diet, it is not really a good diet because it was revealed in a popular magazine.

The *Holiday* business didn't end there. In September of 1951, it published an article by the explorer Earl Parker Hanson that it said had been submitted "unsolicited." Mr. Hanson affirmed the soundness of the diet from his own experience and knowledge. He alluded heavily to what was then known of Eskimos.

*Despite the conviction of many nutritionists that the fat meat diet could not sustain human beings in health over long periods, ethnologists observed that the Eskimos were eating it and seemed, moreover, to be getting a kick out of life—being famous as one of the most laughter-loving peoples on the earth.*

The final article on the subject appeared in *Holiday* in May of 1952, about two years after the first. It was more of an embellishment of the original diet. It mainly added recipes consistent with the principles of the diet. Two years had passed. That was plenty of time for *Holiday* to receive an avalanche of condemnation from an outraged public who had been fooled, had gained weight on their high-calorie meat-and-fat diet, or had suffered severe harm at the hands of such unsound nutritional advice. But apparently, none of that happened. Would a noncontroversial national magazine, not even directed toward nutritional subjects, have continued to advocate a diet that was proving to be harmful?

The presumption is that the positive response that *Holiday* reported was genuine. Yet as with the Banting Diet, interest waned, no significant research was done on the subject, and Pennington was forgotten. He died in 1959.

As in the case of the Banting Diet, no one seemed to say that it didn't work. No one said that Dr. Pennington was falsifying the reports on the weight losses. They did say that the diet was unsound without offering proof of that allegation. Most important of all, they said that the diet should not have been reported in the popular press. It should have been kept in the medical journals.

Curiosity got the best of me, and on March 12, 1991, after some effort, I finally located the doctor's widow. She was a delightful lady, and we had a most interesting telephone conversation. She expresses how to the end Pennington was a staunch believer in his meat diet. She, too, is a believer. She said that she still ate as much meat as she could.

Though meat-and-fat diets seemed to have crossed the Atlantic after Banting's popularity waned, the spark remained and was rekindled in London in 1958. Dr. Richard Mackarness authored *Eat Fat and Grow Slim*, and the world had yet another diet book. You didn't have to get past the preface to know what influenced Mackarness. The preface was written by Evelyn Stefansson, wife of the explorer. It sang the praises of meat and fat and affirmed that this diet was really her husband's diet popularized in England by Mackarness. She confirmed the following:

*The Stone Age all-meat diet is wholesome. It is an eat-all-you-want reducing diet that permits you to forget you are dieting—no hunger pains remind you.*

Mackarness, best known in Britain as a medical writer and columnist, produced the most scholarly book of its type to that date regardless of its suspicious title. He knew the subject well and paid proper British homage to Banting, Pennington, Stefansson, and Donaldson. His diet resembled Pennington's and reiterated one part fat to three parts lean. In defense of this, he echoed a much-shared observation:

*To me, it is inconceivable that fat meat, which has been the staple food of man for millions of years and almost his exclusive food until the introduction of cereal grains six to ten thousand years ago, should suddenly become dangerous because some White Mouse Doctor says so.*

His reference to "White Mouse Doctor" is an obvious dig at the research scientist who derives his knowledge from animal experiments (white mice) rather than from real, live, human patients.

In a long article in the Canadian *Maclean's* magazine in 1959, Dr. Ray N. Lawson, referred to as "a noted Canadian doctor" gave accolades to Mackarness's method and his book. Describing his two years as a "fat-eater," he said, "Not only have I lost the pounds, but I find that I have twice the energy I had before and I have a completely new outlook on life." His article includes before-and-after photos of the then British Conservative party chairman, Lord Hailsham, who surprised his constituents with a massive weight loss on the Mackarness diet. "Meat, all kinds of meat," said Lawson. "And the fatter the better."

If you happened to be an overweight New Yorker during the forties, fifties, or sixties, you might well have been a patient of Blake Donaldson. This controversial physician who practiced at New York

City Hospital, though he did not confine his practice to treating overweight patients, was well known for his interest in the subject. His inclination was that many human problems were associated with nutrition, so his approaches to treating such diverse ailments as osteoarthritis, diabetes, and allergies were not too far from his weight-loss method.

Unashamedly, Dr. Donaldson was a meat lover. Not only did he personally prefer meat, but he felt that a major source of his patients' problems came from the inadequate intake of amino acids that come from a high-grade source of protein such as meat. Furthermore, he was just one more of those advocates of eating meat that was loaded with fat.

Appreciate the fact that he was preaching this doctrine in the fifties and sixties, a period when cholesterol was being recognized as a potential threat to humanity. He was aware of what was being said of fats and cholesterol, and he was very forthcoming in his opposition. His 1961 book, *Strong Medicine,* pretty well states his position. At one point he asks what the reader would do if he were told that he had arteriosclerosis and had recovered from a previous heart attack. Donaldson answered for him:

> *I know what I would do. . . . If I seemed to be overweight I would strive to lose, and if underweight I would strive to gain. Fresh fat meat without salt, potatoes with butter, raw fruit, and black coffee three times a day would be the standard when the body weight is normal. The main consideration in feeding would be the repair of damaged arteries with the fresh fat meat is normal.*

You're probably aware that this is not the kind of nutritional advice your local cardiologist is apt to give his post-coronary patient or even his mildly atherosclerotic one. In fact, he wouldn't give this advice to anyone. But the world has spun around a few times since Donaldson's day, and things have indeed changed.

Has the physical nature of people also changed since that time? If Donaldson's weight-loss diet worked successfully then and produced no harmful effects in his patients, would the same diet work today on, say, you or me? Are we examples of some different organism than the ones he had treated. We know that evolutionary changes do not take place in three generations (and probably not even in 3,000). Is it possible to lose weight by eating quantities of fat meat, or was Donaldson delusional?

He quotes from a letter that he wrote to a particular overweight lady. Maintaining that his patients understand only 5 percent of spoken advice, he liked to put instructions in writing. Thus, he wrote:

> *Your weight is one hundred and ninety pounds. . . . The fastest rate you can expect to lose weight is three pounds a week . . . hundred and seventy-eight consecutive meals, eat nothing but two double rib Frenched lamb chops with pepper on them, and a demitasse of black coffee without sugar. . . . If you are still hungry after eating two chops, you can have as many more as are desired.*

Donaldson was sure rough on his patients. Lamb chops three times a day? I like lamb chops, but there's a limit. From his writing, I picture him as big hearted but gruff. He took a no-nonsense approach with his bizarre method. His further advice to this woman was as follows:

> *Try not to make stupid mistakes. It's too bad if cooking chops at breakfast nauseates you. Just hold your nose. If you lose a meal, go right back at it the next meal.*

Obviously this kind of advice was given during the era when doctors were still treated with uncompromised respect. I couldn't get away with such advice today, no matter how strongly I believed in it. It must have been nice to have such self-assurance.

I have told you these anecdotes about Donaldson to shock you, perhaps to get you out of the rut of your current thinking. You've been influenced strongly by the media. At least understand that, even relatively recently, there have been divergent ideas.

A couple more quotes from Blake Donaldson's book should drive home the point:

> *There may be an upper level of meat intake where no one can lose, but I've never found it.*
>
> . . .
>
> *Most fat people don't eat enough fat meat three times a day to start the fire that will burn off their own excess fat.*

What influenced Donaldson? How did he get started with these ideas? He says that it started with a visit to the Museum of Natural History in New York. He spoke kindly of the curators who allowed him to study the eating habits of primitive peoples, and he decided that the type of diet that allowed them to survive might be just the thing for his own patients.

It should be no surprise that he knew of Stefansson. In fact, he was so anxious to meet the famous man that he entreated a mutual friend to arrange a dinner. Donaldson fed his guest clams and steak and later recounted how he was told stories of the Arctic. He must have been impressed when Stefansson told him of how, after returning to outposts where they could again find groceries, his men still craved the Eskimo diet that they had become accustomed to:

> *A few days of living on the food that they thought would be so wonderful usually finds them back in the Eskimo part of town trying to beg, borrow, or steal some delicious fat from the back of the eyes of the caribou, or else some good seal meat.*

Donaldson's book was not a big success, perhaps because it was just slightly preceded by another diet book that enjoyed tremendous sales and was a difficult act to follow. It doesn't seem that the public can handle two diet books at the same time, and Donaldson had the bad luck to follow immediately on the heels of the book by Brooklyn gynecologist Herman Taller, *Calories Don't Count*.

The book sold very well even though it pushed a diet extremely high in fat. I can't imagine that the readers, eating more than 3,000 calories a day, mostly from fats and oils, albeit "good" oils such as safflower, could have had much success. The book was widely discredited.

The protein diets of the first 100 years or so were essentially inventions of the practitioner who used them. There was little controlled research to prove their effectiveness. The doctors who supervised their patients on these diets knew that they worked because they had front-row seats. To convince others that the diet was effective was often an uphill task. Likewise, the criticism that meat-laced diets came from the seat of someone's pants gave them even less credibility.

A study right out of academia in 1956 was the beginning of change. Two British scientists, Kekwick, a professor at the University of London, and Pawan, from Middlesex Hospital, set out to study the relative effects of carbohydrate, protein, and fat on weight loss in a low-calorie diet.

They selected 14 patients and put them on four different diets in sequence over a period of time. Each of the diets contained 1,000 calories per day, but they differed in the distribution of carbohydrate, protein, and fat. One diet had 90 percent protein, the next, 90 percent fat, the next, 90 percent carbohydrate, and the last was a "normal" mixture of these basic food substances.

Each of the 14 patients was given a period of time on each of the four diets. Since they were hospitalized, they could be monitored for adherence, cheating, etc. The authors admitted that monitoring them was a task. The subjects were not above stealing and getting others to sneak food into the hospital.

In theory, each 1,000 calorie diet should have produced the same weight loss. That is not what happened. The greatest weight loss was on a diet of 90 percent fat. Slightly less weight loss was achieved with 90 percent protein. The mixed diet fell next in the list. The least amount of weight loss was on a 90 percent carbohydrate diet. I have been aware of this study for a long time. Perhaps that explains in part why I have always felt that the craze for diets that are high-carbohydrate (commonly called "complex carbohydrate") in the recent past was completely irrational.

The next part of the experiment was to take five of the group and put them all on the same 2,000 calorie mixed diet for seven days. In this phase, as expected, they pretty well maintained their weights. They were then put on an even higher-calorie diet, 2,600 calories, but composed mostly of fat and protein.

The result was that four out of the five of them lost weight in spite of the fact that they were eating more calories than had maintained them previously on a more balanced diet. Kekwick and Pawan offered the only explanation that they felt was reasonable. Different proportions of carbohydrates, proteins, and fats in the diet alter the metabolism.

It is a shame that the study had not been conducted on a greater number of subjects. Similar results on a larger group would have been more impressive. I imagine that funding was the problem. Still, if a slogan could have been evolved from this study, it might have been "Calories Don't Count." Ironic, isn't it?

This study was possibly the impetus for the proliferation of diets centered on meat. The pace quickened as many doctors jumped on the bandwagon.

Right on the heels of the work of Kekwick and Pawan was a paper authored by George L. Thorpe, MD, chairman of the General Practice section of the American Medical Association. The paper was published as the lead article in the *Journal of the American Medical Association* on November 16, 1957. The journal has always been well respected since it is the scientific voice of the largest physician's organization in the United States. It has never been my impression that *JAMA* publishes diverse points of view unless the opposing view is well founded. This is not meant as criticism. It is simply a journal that presents the mainstream thinking of the moment. That's why I am still surprised not that they published a paper by Dr. Thorpe, but that they published a meat diet. At the time, I had been in practice for only two months and I was so conservative that, *JAMA* or not, I wanted nothing to do with weirdo diets.

Dr. Thorpe summarized his diet in a nice little sidebar at the beginning of the paper. See if any of this sounds familiar:

> *The simplest to prepare and most easily obtainable high-protein, high-fat, low-carbohydrate diet, and the one that will produce the most rapid loss of weight without hunger, weakness, lethargy, or constipation, is made up of meat, fat, and water. The total quantity eaten need not be noted, but the ratio of three part of lean to one part of fat must be maintained. . . . Usually within two or three days, the patient is found to be taking about 170 Gm. of lean meat and 57 Gm. of fat three times a day. Black coffee, clear tea, and water are unrestricted and the salt intake is not reduced. When the patient complains of monotony, certain fruits and vegetables are added for variety.*

Don't bother to do the math, I've already done it. That translates into 2,600 calories per day. His diet sounds like Pennington's, and his results are pretty well consistent with Kekwick and Pawan's. Here was a diet as bizarre as Taller's, printed in a reputable journal rather than in a popular book. I have searched for criticism that could have followed the publication of Thorpe's diet. I could find none.

Let's pause for a moment to reflect on this. Here is a respected AMA member in an honored position who is given considerable space in *JAMA* to state that patients lose weight eating unlimited amounts of meat and fat with no negative effects. The year was 1957, the year I treated my first overweight patient, 52 years ago. If patients lost weight then, would not other patients on that same diet have a similar experience today? I can almost bet that if that very same article were printed today in a popular magazine or in some lesser journal than *JAMA* under a different author's name, it would be mercilessly attacked. Charges would be hurled that not only did the diet not work, it was dangerous.

Banting's country never did lose interest in high-protein diets, though it had to import most of them. But any list of the most authoritative nutritionists of the twentieth century would have to include John Yudkin, MD, of the University of London. In the scientific world, he is known through the hundreds of papers he has written. Among the public on both sides of the Atlantic, he is the curmudgeon who is known as a foe of carbohydrates.

The quintessential carbohydrate is, of course, sugar, and Yudkin's 1972 book, *Sweet and Dangerous*, blasted this commodity like no other ever had. Yudkin had always advocated a low-carbohydrate diet, a fact that has been misinterpreted to mean that he has favored high-protein and high-fat diets. This does not seem to be the case. He simply felt that if you restrict carbohydrates, the whole process will take care of itself.

Dr. Yudkin reported in *The Lancet* in 1960 that he had done studies on some subjects who were instructed to limit their intake of carbohydrates, but to eat as much as they wanted of protein and fat. He observed that they had lost weight, but it was because their total calories were reduced automatically by the restriction of carbohydrate. This came about because, even though told to eat unlimited fat, none of the subjects increased their intake of fat. The implication was that when carbohydrates are reduced, the calorie intake drops also. There is no compensatory increase in the fat intake. In other words, when deprived of carbohydrate, they do not turn to fat as a substitute.

Twelve years later, his paper in *Postgraduate Medicine*, an American journal, told us that he had not altered his position. He called the following instructions a "psychologically impressive statement":

> *You may eat as much as you like of all these foods: meat, fish, eggs, cheese, butter, margarine, oils, cream, leafy vegetables.*

The only food containing fat that was limited was milk, presumably because it also contains considerable carbohydrate.

Yudkin was often quoted by others who advocated low-carbohydrate diets to add credence to their positions. His name was flaunted as if to say, "If Yudkin believes this, it must be true."

A paper published in *JAMA*, written by University of Wisconsin Medical School researchers, reminded one of Taller's diet. "A New Concept in the Treatment of Obesity" described the high-protein, low-carbohydrate diet with which they had achieved success. Except that they broke the meat feedings into six meals, their diet did not seem all that different from Taller's, particularly since it specified the daily use of a quantity of polyunsaturated oil. Another difference between these doctors and Taller was perhaps the fact that, as far as I know, they hadn't written a best-selling book on the subject.

If you ever invent a diet and you want to give it dignity and have it receive proper respect, name it the Air Force Diet. It doesn't matter that it has nothing to do with pilots. You won't get in trouble with our military; they are too busy to worry about such things. The Air Force Diet is what someone named his diet in 1964. I say "someone" because no one seems sure exactly who it was.

Of course, if you would rather have your diet have broad appeal with the "in" crowd, and you're willing to forgo dignity and respect, you could name it the Drinking Man's Diet. That's what Herb Drake did, according to Robert Wernick in a magazine article that was more of a confession. "I Wrote 'The Drinking Man's Diet'" was the title of his declaration. Strangely enough, the 1965 *Saturday Evening Post* article by Wernick says that both diets were essentially the same. Were our brave airmen drinking men?

The Air Force Diet didn't start out as a book. Actually, it first appeared as a few mimeographed sheets that were passed around in business offices. You know how that goes. Sharing interesting or funny material among employees still goes on, but the copy machine and the fax have replaced the mimeograph, and the whole process is much easier today.

For the fashionable crowd, it was a diet sent from above. You could eat all the meat, eggs, butter, and other things you wanted, and you could wash it down with booze. The only restriction was to cut way back on carbohydrates. There went the potatoes, bread, corn, rice, and pasta. Sound familiar?

You did it all by counting carbohydrate grams. No more than 60 per day. Does that sound even more familiar? Today we are still told to do that. We are told to count fat grams. It's the same job with a different focus.

Three enterprising gentlemen, Carroll Lynch, Bob Cameron, and Herb Drake, were said to have commissioned Wernick to rewrite the diet, and in record time, they published it in booklet form. It was the skinniest little nothing of a book you could imagine, but the golden road to getting svelte was sold for a buck apiece, and the public gobbled up *The Drinking Man's Diet*.

I remember seeing one patient after another with this diminutive booklet poking out of a pocket or purse. I imagined then that the authors, Gardner Jameson and Elliott Williams, must have enjoyed tremendous financial success from it, but as it turned out, they hadn't. That's because they didn't exist. The names were phony, and no one seems to know why.

What about the "drinking" part of the diet? Here's the quote from the first page that probably helped sales:

*A diet which allows you to take out your favorite girl for dinner of squab and broccoli with hollandaise sauce and Chateau Lafite, to be followed by an evening of rapture and champagne.*

This page promised more than it delivered because if you read further, you were instructed to limit your drinking considerably.

The book went on to become two Bantam paperbacks, and another American success story was recorded. How was it received? The public reception was great. But the press did not like it nearly as well. *Good Housekeeping* tore it apart in a May 1965 article. Among others, they quoted Dr. Philip L. White of the American Medical Association, well known for his frequent criticism of popular diets and diet books. *Time* magazine also quoted him as saying, "The drinking man's diet is utter nonsense."

Of course, a new diet, like any other new idea, garners respect when it rides the coattails of some respected public figure. Joseph Alsop, the noted political columnist, had only 11 pounds to lose, but to him it was serious business. He did it with the Air Force Diet, which he insisted, although not officially sanctioned by them, had close ties with the Air Force. So delighted was he with losing his weight by simply limiting himself to between 40 and 60 grams of carbohydrate per day, he sang the praises of this diet in *McCall's* in a May 1965 article. His paperback book account of the same diet, *Drink, Eat, and Be Thin,* expressed his gratitude to the diet that he called his "gift from heaven." I could find no mention in either his article or his book of the Drinking Man's Diet.

Of course, now that I have made you into a skeptic, you may wonder whether Alsop's accolades for the diet could have been a scheme to sell books. That is hardly the case. A writer with his credentials doesn't need to prostitute himself to sell a few paperbacks. He was just so pleased with his new body that he sincerely wanted to share his good fortune with his fellow man.

Whether it was the nonsense that Dr. White believed it to be or not, the public, after more than 100 years, was continuing to support the high-protein, low-carbohydrate method of losing weight. Is it really possible that some universal delusion such as this on the part of the doctors and their patients or subjects such as Alsop could really continue for such an extended period?

An article entitled "Diet of Whipped Cream" in *Science News Letter* in 1965 must have attracted some attention. It reviewed a presentation given by Dr. Broda O. Barnes before a session of the Federation of American Societies for Experimental Biology. He advocated, like some others, a diet low in carbohydrate and a moderate amount of protein but high in fat. Barnes's diet was a marvel. For breakfast he suggested two eggs, three strips of bacon, and a small, peeled orange. The high point came later. Every four hours his patients ate nothing but a drink consisting of one pint of whipping cream, one egg, artificial sweetener, vanilla, and nutmeg. An abstract of his presentation adds succinctly, "No heart attacks have occurred during the use of diets rich in saturated fats for over 25 years."

Barnes was another critic of the cholesterol-heart connection (obviously), but his major cause had to do with metabolism and the thyroid gland. I share his interest in that subject. I'll talk about that in Chapter 14.

In the sixties diets and diet books exploded on the scene. Gayelord Hauser, the popular food columnist, who had told us in the fifties in *New Guide to Intelligent Reducing* to lose it with lots of lean meat and healthful but limited fruits and vegetables, repeated his advice in *The New Diet Does It*. A Louisville internist, Dr. Irving B. Perlstein said you have to build your diet around meat because "the more lean meat you eat, the more weight you will lose." He was a believer in the specific dynamic action of protein that was mentioned earlier in this chapter. *The L-C Diet* (low carbohydrate) that he purported to be "widely known as the low carbohydrate Air Force diet" was obviously attempting to ride the heels of the Drinking Man's success.

Everyone knew who Carlton Fredericks was because his name was universally associated with nutritional advice. In *Dr. Carlton Fredericks' Low-Carbohydrate Diet and Eat-More-to-Lose-More Diet Book*, he advocated a lot of small meals a day, but they should be full of meat and with considerable fat. He said that carbohydrates were "the real mischief-makers." Another nutritional activist, Sidney Petrie, though not a physician, said he treated lots of overweight people in his Long Island office. He seemed to turn out a diet book about once a year. Take your pick: you can follow *The Lazy Lady's Easy Diet, How to Reduce and Control Your Weight through Self-Hypnotism*, or attack your fat with *Fat Destroyer Foods*. My favorite title of his was *Martinis and Whipped Cream*. Like many others, he said to eat protein and meat and cut carbohydrates to a minimum. He maintained that eating fat was an absolute necessity when on a high-protein diet.

Another try at a diet that allowed alcohol was Dr. Ernest R. Reinsh's, *Eat, Drink, and Get Thin*, published in 1969. He was more opposed to carbonated drinks than he was to liquor. He allowed one "shot of Bourbon, Scotch, Rye, Gin, or Vodka." As to beef, "Pile it on." How about butter? "All you want." Lard, margarine, oil? He advocated the same. But for carbohydrates, he advised to eat very little.

In the 1970s some showbiz people started passing out weight-losing advice. Naura Hayden, a budding television actress, wrote *The Hip, High-Prote, Low-Cal, Easy-Does-It Cookbook*. A real "name" was Ed McMahon, who sat right next to Johnny Carson on *The Tonight Show* and who was constantly kidded about his drinking. McMahon wrote *Slimming Down* to inform the world of his weight-losing success. Although McMahon talks about the Drinking Man's Diet, he gives full credit for his weight loss to Sidney Petrie's book *Martinis and Whipped Cream*. You can probably guess which of those two "diet foods" he preferred. McMahon liked Petrie's "carbo-calorie" charts, which were simply lists of foods with their carbohydrate grams multiplied by four, the number of calories in each gram of carbohydrate. Another book, *The Carbo-Calorie Diet* by Donald S. Mart, seemed to also take credit for the carbo-calorie concept.

Even U.S. senators had trouble resisting the urge to write diet books. Senator William Proxmire wrote *You Can Do It!* in 1973, but his method had more to do with exercise than it did with diet.

Books by doctors always carried more respect. Dr. Irwin Maxwell Stillman was such a lovable gent that you just had to trust his diet. Since I never had the pleasure of meeting him, how did I know he was lovable? The answer is because I saw him so frequently on television talk shows that I felt I knew him.

He was a cute little fellow with an acid wit who could delight an audience such as that of *The Tonight Show*. He and Johnny Carson would parry and thrust, and the audience loved it. There he pitched his diet and his book masterfully.

*The Doctor's Quick Weight Loss Diet* describes not just one diet, but such a multitude of options that one could lose weight from not eating while trying to decide which diet to follow.

Stillman, who did not like being called a "diet doctor," insisted that he was a retired family doctor who had perfected a weight-loss diet that worked miracles on 12,000 of his patients back in Brooklyn.

Stillman differed sharply with many of the "high-protein men" in that he did not want his patients eating fat. On many of his diets, you could have all the lean meat, fish, eggs, and low-fat cheese you wanted; carbohydrates were kept to a minimum, consistent with the advice of every other proponent of high-protein living. Actually he wasn't all that consistent when you realize the high fat content of eggs. "Eight glasses of water a day" was practically his signature phrase.

So great was the success of the Stillman Diet that the publishers probably lost track of the number of printings of his paperback. They hungered for more and he obliged. *The Doctor's Quick Weight-Loss Diet* was followed by *The Doctor's Quick Weight-Loss Diet Cookbook, The Doctor's Quick Inches-Off Diet, The Doctor's Quick Teenage Diet, Dr. Stillman's 14-Day Shape-up Program,* and on and on it went. There were innumerable paperback spin-offs and translations, and there seemed to be such a frenzy to translate them into other languages that you can probably find Stillman in languages that have long been extinct.

What did the critics think of Stillman? What would you expect? He was actually treated somewhat better than many of his colleagues who had written diet books. The criticism was strongest when it came to cholesterol. A group from Harvard published a paper in 1974 in *JAMA* on how Stillman's diet affected cholesterol. Noting that 5 million people bought his original book, they decided to test the diet for a couple of weeks on 12 hospital employees. They reported a significant average increase in serum cholesterol in the group. Thus, they concluded that the diet posed "potential risks." Incidentally, the group of 12 averaged seven pounds of weight loss.

If 5 million bought the book, you have to guess that the last two and a half million of those must have bought it as a result of someone's recommendation or because of its notoriety. I somehow don't remember any public outcry stemming from any "damage" to 5 million people exposed to "potential risk." In fact, I've never heard of a single case, although I allow for the fact that someone, somewhere, must have complained of harm.

When Stillman died, so did the charisma, but his books didn't die. You can still find them in the bookstores.

Another practicing physician to question the belief that a calorie is a calorie was George Schauf, M.D., of California. In an article in *Nutrition Today* in 1971 entitled "All Calories Don't

Count…Perhaps," he said that he allowed his patients an egg, bacon, buttered toast, and coffee with cream for breakfast. Lunch and dinner consisted of meat with minimal carbohydrates but a required amount of polyunsaturated oil. He said, "By shifting the diet toward more protein and fat and away from carbohydrate, we can have patients who do not get abnormally hungry, who retain ample energy, and who are apt to continue the regimen prescribed."

Schauf strengthened and reiterated his position two years later in the *Journal of the American Geriatrics Society*, citing research that indicated that carbohydrates favor the depositing of fat on the body, while fat in the diet increases lipolysis, or removal of stored fat. He obviously couldn't resist joining the ranks of diet book authors. *Think Thin* in 1976 rehashed the whole thing.

The year 1972 was a big year for diet books. That's when the *Boston Police Diet* was hot. It would have been hotter if it hadn't been for Dr. Atkins's great success at that same time. Its author, Sam Berman, a practicing medical doctor, claimed that at the time of writing the book, the program had been used by some 400 participants from the Boston Police Department. He said it worked.

Berman generally followed the party line of Pennington. Allowing a bit more variety, he advocated all kinds of meat for breakfast and dinner and sardines, tuna, or salmon for lunch. His position on dietary fat seems unclear to me. On the one hand, he allowed such things as lobster dipped in melted butter, fried foods, skin of chicken or turkey, and whipped cream. Yet he suggests draining the oil from tuna or sardines.

*Fat as a specific food group, has the highest caloric value of the three food groups.* But fats are not fattening. *Because they have more than double the amount of calories found in the other two groups*, fats represent the greatest source of potential energy and heat.

He went on to say the following:

> *The BPD Program doesn't restrict fats, per se. If you like some fat on your meat, or from other sources . . . help yourself. Enjoy!*

He advised against refined sugars but allows fruits that contain sugar. He said no to cereal, ice cream, sweetened beverages, jellies, jams, preserves, rice, potatoes, corn, beans, beets, parsnips, sweetened yogurt, alcoholic beverages, bread, batter, things made with flour, and most fruits.

If there was any real distinction between Dr. Berman's diet and the others, it is this: he stated very clearly that the diet works best when taken with "The Supplement." Although the supplement is mentioned repeatedly, you have to work to discover what it is. Eventually he identified it but only once by name. If you missed that line, you were out of luck. The supplement is the hormone of the thyroid gland.

Berman must have had some unresolved conflict when it came to thyroid as an adjunct to his program. His cat-and-mouse references to it were quite mysterious. Since his supplement required a prescription, the reader needed the family doctor's cooperation.

The Boston Police Diet was just one more of those diets that gave the individual the license to pig out on steak, hamburgers, bacon, and eggs. Berman really liked eggs. "I eat an average of four eggs daily," he freely admitted.

What was the result of all this? If we are to believe Berman, 400 svelte and happy Irish cops patrolling the streets of Beantown.

The prize for the most controversial of all the diet book authors might very well go to Dr. Robert C. Atkins. If you were to read his 1972 *Dr. Atkins' Diet Revolution* along with a dozen or so of the books we have already mentioned, it would not be apparent that he should be singled out for special treatment. His book is, in fact, better organized and presented than most of the others. His approach is clear enough, though the justification is cloudy yet no more obscure than for any diet, even the so-called accepted diets. The truth is that we don't know an awful lot about nutrition. It's difficult to theorize about any diet.

It seems that there have always been two camps when it comes to diet. There is the conventional group who are made up of the esteemed members of the medical establishment who brandish credentials from respected learning institutions, organizations, or even the government's health-oriented services. It is automatically assumed that they know what they are talking about. Although they claim effectiveness for their methods, their main focus is to convince us that their methods are "safe," whereas others are not. Their approaches might be dubbed "conventional" diets.

The conventional people promulgate their advice. Obviously some of the overweight public follow it and lose weight. Few follow the advice for very long, and thus, they regain. The recidivism rate is characterized as a national disgrace. Their cry is, "We give you good advice. Why don't you take it?"

They are right and they are wrong. If taken, their advice would work. But the public is reluctant to take the advice. The result is that people lose a little weight then gain at least that amount back. The problem is, therefore, assigned to the public, never to the advice. Is there anything familiar here? Have you ever given anyone good advice only to have your well-meaning effort rejected? In particular, has this ever happened with your own children?

In dealing with excess weight, we are dealing with a major health problem affecting millions. Unless the nutritional advice given is the kind that people are willing to accept, it doesn't help any more than bad or erroneous advice would. It is essentially useless. Its value is principally to the advice-giver, who can pompously declare, "I've told you the right thing to do. If you don't follow my advice, that's your problem."

The other side of the coin belongs to the "radical" advice-givers. They have discovered that there are alternative ways to accomplish the goal of losing weight. They have observed that certain types of diets are more apt to be followed than those of the conventional diet gurus. They, like their conventional counterparts, espouse theories for why their diets work, and they make no more sense than any others. Their efforts are really frantic attempts to explain the unknown, an activity rather common to mankind. They, like the conventionalists, know that their methods work, are equally frustrated in their ability to explain why they do, but do have the knowledge that their diets are better received by the public.

That, I believe, is the state of dietary treatment. For the most part, the diet proponents chronicled so far in this book have been the radical, the unconventional, those who have observed that their methods work better and are more apt to be followed. The conventionalists are understandably hostile and have the added advantage of having the "ear" of the media. They are able to freely wage their battle through printed and electronic information. The radical people are less apt to get their message across gratis, and they rely heavily on paid advertising to tell their story. The public tends to believe news stories in favor of paid ads, so the radicals are generally regarded as suspect. So the battle goes on between the conventional and the unconventional. What tilts the balance is the fact that the conventional group determines who belongs in their group.

In the end it gets very confusing. The unconventional (high-protein) group seems to outnumber the conventional. Perhaps the titles should be reversed.

My little discourse on conventionality and unconventionality fits well into our look at Atkins because he, more than any of the others, was singled out to represent what was bad about the radical approach to dieting.

According to Atkins, he was a practicing cardiologist in Manhattan who one day found that he was too fat. Not willing to accept the current regimens, he did some library research to search for a better way. He discovered Pennington, Donaldson, and probably others whom I have already mentioned. He says he was particularly influenced by a paper written by Drs. Bloom and Azar in *The Archives of Internal Medicine* in 1963. Atkins tells us that he was impressed that subjects on a total fast and subjects on a diet devoid of carbohydrate shared a common finding—the absence of hunger.

He put himself on what he called "Bloom's diet" but gradually increased his carbohydrate allowance to 40 grams. At this level, he lost weight consistently and had no hunger. He described how he ate frequent snacks, "cheese, cold cuts, cold shrimp, cottage cheese." High protein was the rule, fat content was largely ignored, but it was important to ingest little carbohydrate.

The whole thing was organized into a book that became one of the all-time diet best-sellers. Atkins truly had little to add to what has already been said here, but his program was packaged nicely; the book was easy to read, and the public bought it.

Before Atkins's book came out in paperback, *Lose Pounds the Low-Carbohydrate Way* by Myra Waldo was published. The cover screamed, "Why wait for Dr. Atkins' Diet Revolution? Here now, in paperback . . ." Imitation is indeed the sincerest compliment.

The onslaught on Atkins was tremendous. He was harangued from every quarter. Denunciations appeared in the most reputable of medical publications. Whereas most diet books barely get a one-column review in *JAMA*, Atkins's book deserved a five page rebuke that even included 56 citations to other sources, presumably that advanced *JAMA*'s point of view. To present their objections in a nutshell, the diet was dangerous, particularly because of the fats, which increased "the risk of coronary artery disease."

The article attacked Atkins in particular by attacking unconventional diets in general:

*Moreover, despite the claims of universal and painless success for such diets, no nationwide decrease in obesity has been reported.*

How do you interpret this remark? Are they hinting that the conventional diets have produced such a "nationwide decrease in obesity?" Are they telling us that "such diets" as Atkins's have been given a nationwide scientific trial and simply didn't work. Furthermore, the article spoke of "potential hazards" but did not cite one single case of known harm from it. What was truly lacking was any clear-cut statement to the effect that persons following this diet do not lose weight. The absence of such a declaration seems counterproductive to the article's objectives. It gives tacit confirmation that the diet does work.

Seven months later, a well-known name from Harvard University Medical School replied to a reader's query in *JAMA*. Though still very negative toward Atkins and his "erroneous science and logic," he did seem to admit that this type of diet "appears to effect a weight reduction."

Atkins wrote more diet books and continued to practice in New York until his death in a freak accident in 2003. He seemed always to be in and out of the news. One day in April of 1993, 21 years after his big splash, I watched his crucifixion. It seems that he had recently written a new diet book. He was obviously anxious to get public exposure. He accepted an invitation to appear on *Geraldo* and walked into a trap. He arrived, well armed, book in hand, with an entourage of patients who were there to confirm the value of his method and to spout testimonials. His own wife was there along with some of his employees.

In an introduction to the show, Geraldo Rivera flashed his book, and if you listened carefully, you might have picked up that a new diet book was around. Someone might have gotten in a quick plug. That was the end of the discussion of reducing diets. There was no more talk of weight loss or of his books. Apparently the show knew that Atkins had branched out into other fields of "alternative medicine." He was ambushed. The rest of the hour paraded experts who demolished his treatment methods. They zoomed in on former patients who told their horror stories. He was lambasted for making too much money. Atkins weakly sputtered his defenses, but he was hopelessly unprepared to defend against the surprise attack. He was there to talk about diet, but they weren't interested in diet. That was simply not the topic of the day. He reminded me of General Custer, although Atkins did manage to get out alive—barely.

The criticisms of high-protein diets have often alluded to potential harm but have rarely documented actual harm. This was not the case of the liquid protein fiasco of the seventies. The origins of the diet could probably be traced to Dr. Alan Howard in England or perhaps to Dr. George Blackburn in Boston. They seemed to believe that a semifasting type of diet would be acceptable in certain individuals if they would receive sufficient protein to prevent muscle wasting. It had been observed that complete fasting resulted in not only fat loss, but also a certain amount of muscle loss, which was quite undesirable, particularly if the muscle was in some vital structure, such as the heart.

Thus, some proposed very-low-calorie diets that would supply enough protein to avoid this effect. The term *protein-sparing modified fast* was coined. Someone had the bright idea that the protein could best be drunk rather than eaten, and almost overnight the stores were full of "liquid protein," a rather distasteful beverage made essentially from the hides of cattle. Its constituents, the amino acids of protein, were similar to those of gelatin but shared the latter's deficiency of certain of these amino acids. In order for a protein to be rated as "high quality," it must have a certain proportionate mixture of its basic constituents, the amino acids. The liquid product was indeed protein but a very substandard form of it. It did not compare in quality with the kind of protein found in milk, eggs, fish, foul, or meat. The use of these products as the sole source of food became a national fad as well as a national disaster when a number of deaths were reported among those who had been on these exclusively liquid-protein diets. Obviously a diet of just any protein was not a proper substitute for the meat that had been the backbone of the human diet for so many years.

There were theories as to why these deaths occurred, but the exact mechanism was never clearly defined. Still, it seemed logical that this inferior mixture of amino acids was implicated in some way, understood or not, and liquid protein vanished from the scene as quickly as it appeared.

Atkins's diet was untouched by this interlude and stayed popular throughout the eighties, but the crown was eventually passed out of the Big Apple to the suburbs and to Herman Tarnower, MD. *The Complete Scarsdale Medical Diet* was published in 1979. Its popularity didn't last as long as the diet that preceded it, perhaps because it was more vague than Atkins's diet. Though more than one diet was described in his book, Tarnower featured a "14-Day Diet," which I seem to recall was the more popular. He also pushed meat, "plenty of broiled steak, all visible fat removed," but minimal fat and moderate carbohydrate. He also believed that protein was the key to weight loss, stating that his diet contained triple the amount of protein as did the typical American diet. The book said little that was innovative. A review of diets by the editors of *Consumer Guide* found it "foolish and forgettable" and dubbed it "Stillman's Ghost."

The mid-eighties were a dry period for "meat" diets, which was understandable. The National Cholesterol Education Program was launched, and meat was "out." Yet in 1988 *The Paleolithic Prescription*, a quite scholarly popular book was published. The authors, Eaton, Shostak, and Konner, were from the academic world. Eaton was a radiologist, and his co-authors, professors of anthropology.

Their prescription was to return to the general eating and exercise habits of the Stone Age people. It was shades of Stefansson, whom, surprisingly, they did not mention. They recognized meat as a primary source of prehistoric human food, but their estimates of how many carbohydrates were eaten was in excess of what most of the authorities quoted previously had believed. This was probably because they used as their yardstick the diet of present-day "Stone Age" people. Recognizing that today's Stone Agers have diets that vary with their regions of the world (e.g., perhaps 90 percent animal food for Eskimos but only 20 percent for Australian Aborigines), they tried to strike a balance by averaging. They concluded that the number of calories derived from carbohydrate, protein, and fat should be in the ration of 3:1:1.

The book, although not a weight-loss book as such, but rather a "prescription" for healthy living, did touch on reducing but rather obliquely. If you one day find yourself fat, they advise that you do what your ancestors did. "Create a temporary food shortage by reducing caloric intake and increasing physical exertion." Though I disagreed with many of their conclusions, I liked the book and would recommend it.

Not exactly a "meat diet" book but one that did allow meat twice a day in moderate amounts was the 1991 *The Carbohydrate Addict's Diet*. Drs. Richard and Rachael Heller were medical school professors, though not physicians. They highlight what they call a carbohydrate "addiction" and advise two meals a day of very low carbohydrate. Their approach is novel, but in reading their well-meaning advice, I cannot help but conclude that their knowledge is academic and does not seem to flow from the experience of actually treating many overweight patients. Still, their book demonstrates that even into the nineties, high-protein, low-carbohydrate diets were not dead.

From about 1990 to the present, there has been an impressive quantity of new diet books. Everyone was jumping on the bandwagon. And why not? Obesity was increasing at an alarming rate.

I've devoted a lot of space to the various doctors' diets over the years. They fascinated me. Until very recently, the emphasis was on protein. In the nineties the shift away from protein was obvious and the incidence of obesity skyrocketed.

With that quantity of new books to comment on, you should logically be in for a lot more pages of commentary from me. Relax. I have little more to say because those books had little more to say. Except to ridicule some really way-out and obviously stupid concepts, there was absolutely nothing new on which to comment. Some that should be mentioned are the following:

There was a book by Dean Ornish, MD, in 1993 that was a tribute to carbohydrates. His claim was that his diet was good for your heart. It might be good if it really got the weight off. I found nothing to suggest hunger control, especially with all those carbs.

Dr. Barry Sears, PhD, and his *The Zone Diet* (1995) seemed to have a good following. His diet was low calorie and emphasized protein. I must agree. But how about hunger?

*The Paleo Diet* (2002) by Loren Cordain, PhD, while not exactly new, was somewhat interesting. Eat like your ancestors. That brought back memories of Stefansson and a well-written 1988 book by three obviously well-educated people, *The Paleolithic Prescription*. (I believe Siegal had a bit to say about that type of diet.)

Medical doctor Arthur Agatston's *South Beach Diet* (2003) was certainly the biggest financial success, but I'm not sure why. Like many diets, it would work if the dieter weren't hungry and if the weight loss were speedy enough to maintain one's motivation.

Sorry, I didn't review *Skinny Bitch* (2005).

Oh, I forgot to mention *Dr. Siegal's Cookie Diet Book*. You ought to read it.

# Section Three

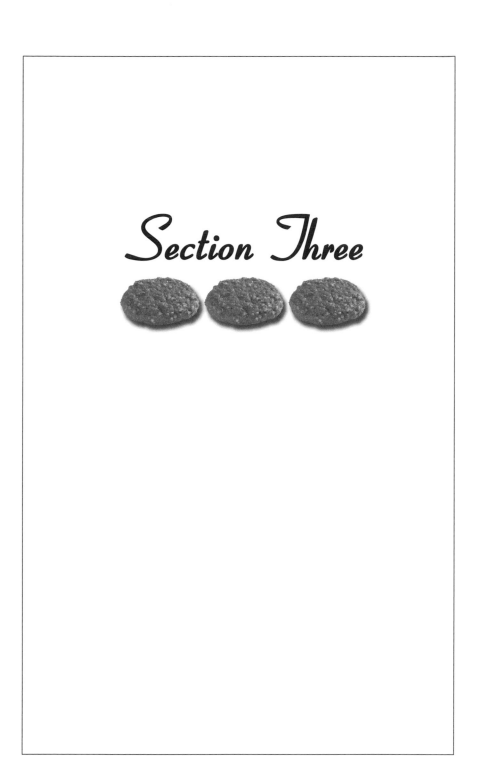

*Chapter 12*

# The Great Calorie Theory

There are lots of diets. And there are lots of nutritionists and lots of doctors who fancy themselves as experts in the field. There are lots of researchers who toil to find clues to the puzzle of excess weight, and there are even a fair amount of theories as to the actual mechanism by which we lose and gain weight.

There's very little that's consistent among the experts concerning the broad theories of how the whole thing happens. Yet at least for the last 200 years, they have been rather consistent as to the basic explanation. Virtually everyone believes in The Great Calorie Theory. I'm included in the believers but maybe not quite 100 percent.

Have you ever heard of The Great Calorie Theory? No? Of course not. That's because I just invented the name. Not the theory, mind you. I didn't invent that. I just invented the name. It's difficult to continually refer to a complicated explanation of how something happens if it doesn't have a name. So for the purpose of this book, in fact, maybe only this chapter, you'll know what I mean each time I refer to The Great Calorie Theory. When you've finished this book, you can conveniently forget that name because no one ever calls it that. It's even possible that you may choose to forget what the The Great Calorie Theory represents. It's OK with me.

If you've read any of my previous books, please don't embarrass me by pointing out that I have never questioned the theory before. We all have to grow, don't we?

Actually it may not even be a *theory*. The definition of *theory* suggests that it's a group of ideas that fit together to explain how some phenomenon occurs. Scientists differentiate among such things as axioms, principles, rules, and hypotheses, and indeed The Great Calorie Theory may actually be one of these. But this is not a book about semantics. As long as we both know what I'm talking about, The Great Calorie Theory will do just fine. Now let's get on with it.

What makes it "great"? The Great Calorie Theory (TGCT) is so universal in its acceptance that any new ideas about diet always operate within the ground rules of TGCT. It seems no one ever questions it. This might be analogous to a discussion group within a church arguing about why God does this or does that, but no one in that group questions the existence of God. That God exists is simply accepted. Any doubter would probably not be in that group to begin with. What makes TGCT "great" is that it is so universally accepted.

Indeed, as you read this book, you'll probably have the impression that I accept TGCT unequivocally. That's because the dogma attached to it is good enough to be the basis for a set of instructions for losing weight that really works. It's "good enough," but don't get the idea that I'm saying it's perfect.

We've been told, *ad nauseam*, that our weights are controlled by the number of calories that we take in (eat) counterbalanced by the number of calories that we use, or "burn."

I'll remind you that strictly speaking, a calorie is really a unit of energy as defined by scientists. It is actually heat energy.

Furthermore, what we really call a calorie is truly 1,000 calories, or what scientists call a kilocalorie. So when we speak of calories, we really mean kilocalories. But in this book, to avoid confusing you with the truth, I'll use *calorie* to mean what you've always believed it to mean, and that is that number that appears opposite "broccoli" in that little book you bought.

When we eat, we take in calories, energy. If our little book tells us how many calories are in such things as a floret of broccoli or a teaspoon of sugar, with a little effort and a pocket calculator, we can add up the calories in everything we've eaten in the course of a day.

There are also books that purport to tell us how many calories our bodies burn in a day. They do this by suggesting that all of us burn up a certain "basal" amount by just existing. It has never been clear to me whether this basal state occurs when I'm in a coma or just sitting in a chair watching television, two activities that may not be all that different. Nonetheless, numbers are given for both men and women since they differ in terms of calorie use. We must then add to this basal amount the number of calories that is consumed by each activity in which we indulge. If the book says that brushing your teeth uses up 35 calories, that must be added to your basal calorie use.

At any rate, you can come up with a number that represents how many calories you've burned during a particular day. It must be obvious that if we are to use those printed guidelines to calculate our calorie usage, it would be nice if they were accurate. Yet we don't all brush our teeth for the same length of time or with the same enthusiasm, and there must be marked differences in how many calories are used while brushing. Besides, I challenge those who supply us with this information to validate their accuracy by telling us how and where they got their information. Did they really observe subjects while diagnostic machines were attached to them as they performed their daily dental hygiene? The idea that we use a specified number of calories to perform each little function does, however, make for nice, neat little calorie books.

So we add up how many calories we eat during a particular day and subtract how many calories we've burned during that day to discover that there was either an excess or deficit of calories.

For example:

| | |
|---|---|
| Total calories eaten | 3,250 |
| Total calories burned | 2,250 |
| Excess calories | 1,000 |

Here we've eaten 1,000 calories more than was burned. The Great Calorie Theory tells us that for each 3,500 calories that we eat over what we burn, we gain one pound in the form of stored fat. That's because the calorie content of a pound of fat is 3,500 calories. It's supposedly true for all fats. This number applies to fat such as cooking oil and also to the type of fat that's in your body. Actually both these fats are really somewhat more than 3,500 calories per pound, but it will not be profitable to explain the discrepancy since, as you have already guessed, we are warming up to attack the theory in its entirety.

So eating 1,000 calories more than you burn will cause you to gain a little less than one-third of a pound. If you were to eat that exact same excess every day, you would gain about one-third of a pound every single day. TGCT says that that would amount to more than 120 pounds in a year. That would be an impressive weight gain in one year! And in 10 years, that would amount to 1,200 pounds!

Here is where The Great Calorie Theory fails. I'm not aware of anyone alive today who weighs 1,200 pounds more than his normal weight. He would have to weigh 1,300 or more pounds. There are people who daily eat thousands of calories more than they burn and who have been doing so for many years.

In terms of the opposite scenario, losing weight, were you to eat 1,000 calories less in a day than you use up, you would be expected to lose one-third of a pound each day. It's not likely that you could continue doing this for a year unless you were really tremendously overweight to begin with, for you would be expected to lose 120 pounds during that year. Of course, there are people who need to lose that much. In January 2009, a woman who lost 120 lbs (half her body weight!) on Dr. Siegal's Cookie Diet was featured on the cover of *People* magazine.

These various scenarios should alert you to the fact that all is not rosy with The Great Calorie Theory. To a certain extent, TGCT does explain why we get fat or why we lose weight. We certainly know that the amount and type of food eaten has a lot to do with the problem. We also know that the activities that we indulge in are another factor. Both of these are obvious contributors to our weights. But the absolute confidence that the scientific community and the public have in TGCT appears to me to be suspect.

Actually the public may not be all that confident that The Great Calorie Theory is valid. If my own patients are anything like a cross-section of the overweight public, they don't seem to buy the theory on faith. A day doesn't go by that some patient doesn't say to me, "I don't overeat, yet I'm overweight." Or, "If on one day, I go off the diet and eat a few extra calories, I gain several pounds." According to TGCT, he or she would have to have eaten 3,500 extra calories for each pound gained.

I've had to deal with this kind of thing day in and day out for many years. My approach has been rather rigid. I'm not one to tamper with the laws of the universe. Believing that The Great Calorie Theory was one of those universal truths, I've had to evaluate each paradoxical uttering by each patient on an individual basis in order to explain away the obvious paradox. I would decide that Patient A had a lower metabolism than our laboratory results indicated. Patient B was mistaken. She was deluding herself. She really didn't realize how much she was eating. Besides, her arithmetic was bad. Patient C clearly needed to buy a new bathroom scale. And as far as Patient D was concerned, he was just a plain liar. That took care of him.

While all this was going on, I must confess that a very uncomfortable feeling dogged me. Who was I to pass judgment on such earnest supplications of so many people? I sat in judgment like some superior being. I didn't feel that I had any alternative. TGCT said that what was being reported to me was impossible, and we all know that the impossible isn't really possible.

What, then, could be wrong with The Great Calorie Theory? Was it totally wrong? Was it only partly wrong? Was it right for some people and wrong for others? Was it right for certain classes of foods and wrong for others? Should it be modified or junked? What could explain why all the "experts" have such faith in TGCT, yet my faith in it is shaky and, I suspect, so is that of perhaps millions of others. The public is less inclined to have faith in TGCT than are the respected experts. The point is that I'm a professional; I'm supposed to profit by the millions of dollars spent in research. I'm supposed to accept what the people in the ivory towers have passed down to me. But I can't always. I've seen with my own eyes that "it ain't necessarily so."

We're not going to truly answer any of these questions in this book. It will take much interest, time, money, labor, and enthusiasm before questions such as these are answered. But I am going to offer some observations.

Let's recapitulate. If The Great Calorie Theory is reliable, then logic tells us that there should be more than a few 1,300 or 1,500 pound people out there. But where are they? I haven't seen a single one. Have you?

Earlier I gave you this very example of what might happen, under TGCT, if a person were to eat an extra 1,000 calories per day. There would be an enormous weight gain over the long haul. But what would happen if someone were to eat only 100 extra calories per day. A single orange can have that number of calories. The weight gain would only be 10 percent of what was calculated earlier. Thus, in 10 years there would be a gain of 120 pounds over the starting weight. To dramatize it, a 120 pound woman who carefully tried to eat the exact amount of calories that would maintain her weight but who erred and actually ate the equivalent of an extra orange each day would end up weighing 240 pounds in 10 years. After 20 years, she would be 360 pounds! Do you think that there are people out there who have the best of intentions but still miss the mark by, say, one extra orange per day? That shouldn't be too hard to accept.

What's wrong with my scenario relating to this lady is that we can't really know how many calories she's eating. The *exact* information isn't available to us. The U.S. Department of Agriculture does a good job of trying to supply us with this data. They continually revamp their databases with the latest up-to-date information on the calorie counts of all known foods. Yet if, for example, one of their tables should tell us that a medium orange with a diameter of three inches contains in its edible portion 73 calories, can we rely upon it?

What is *edible* for you may not be what is edible for me, and both can differ from what is edible to the researcher who tested the oranges. But what difference should that make? Suppose one person eats a little more of the pulp than another. What difference do such a few calories make? Anyway, when is the last time you measured an orange with a ruler before you ate it? Do you know that the table says that a medium orange containing 73 calories is said to measure three inches across. The same table says that a large orange, which measures three-eighths of an inch more, has 115 calories. Try to measure the diameter of an orange with a ruler and you'll appreciate the difficulty in assessing how many calories it contains.

This same line of inquiry could extend to most foods. I've even touched on the fact that agricultural products are not standardized. A three-inch orange grown during one year may not have the same calorie count as an identical-sized orange of another year. And California oranges differ from Florida oranges. We know that grapes vary from year to year; that's why there are such vast differences in the price of wines of different vintages. Furthermore, agricultural produce can vary according to the time of year they are grown or because of the location of the farm.

What I'm telling you is that you must, even in this area of assessing the calories you are eating, become an informed skeptic, or you will be spinning your wheels, making senseless calculations that have no validity.

A moment ago I asked what difference an error of a few calories would make. The answer is a lot. How else are you going to stay at a proper weight? I doubt that in our ordinary assessment of what we eat we can come within 25 percent of the true number. If such small alterations in the number of calories consumed can make such a difference in what you weigh over an extended period, it becomes essential that you know *exactly* how many calories you're eating. Otherwise, why deceive yourself? Why waste your time?

We're not done with this subject. Until now we've spoken only of how many calories were in the foods we've eaten. But is it the food that actually goes into your mouth that counts? Let's look closer. What happens if you chew up your food and spit it out? Obviously you would get some of the calories to drop into your stomach but not all of them. The same would be true for the bulimic person who eats then forces herself to throw up. Do you think that if you swallow a quantity of food, you get every last calorie of that food to nourish your body? Certainly not. A certain amount of food passes right through your body and is expelled when you have a bowel movement. I'll try not to be indelicate. What's in the toilet has calories, the ones you didn't get.

Why isn't every last calorie used? There are a number of reasons. The speed by which the food passes through your stomach and intestinal tract has much to do with it. Different parts of your food are *digested* in different sections of the long passage. Digestion is the chemical process by which the food you eat is chemically changed into the components that can be absorbed into your bloodstream. Digestion is necessary before your body can actually use the food or the calories contained in it. You can't, for example, crush up an apple, put it into a syringe, and inject it directly into your bloodstream. Take my word for it; no good would come from it. Let's be a little more explicit; it would kill you. It has to be digested first in that long tube that starts with your lips and ends up quite a distance south.

If your food passes through you at a very rapid rate, less of it is digested and absorbed because there wouldn't be enough time for these processes to take place. Many things influence how fast your food goes through you, and it happens faster in some than in others. Illness is certainly one of these influences. Diarrhea is an example of superfast transit of food through your digestive tract with diminished use of the calories it contains. I once wrote a book[1] that claimed that a lot of fiber in your diet made your food move a lot faster.

Another reason you don't digest all your food is because the enzymes, chemicals that act upon the food to digest it, might not be able to make physical contact with the food. Without getting too graphic, have you ever suspected that the corn on the cob you had eaten yesterday was not thoroughly digested? If you happened to note that some kernels made it out of your body relatively intact, it's obvious that you didn't get the benefit of the calories contained in those particular kernels. Thus, when you went to record that ear of corn in your calorie diary for the day, you should probably have subtracted the calories from the kernels that survived the trip through your intestines.

---

[1] *Dr. Siegal's Natural Fiber Permanent Weight-Loss Diet* (The Dial Press, 1975)

I haven't included all the reasons you can't accurately count your calorie intake, but I hope that by now you see the impossibility of truly getting it right.

Let's go back now and remember that as far as what contributes to what you weigh, calorie intake is only half of the story. The other half is the energy we expend. If you think measuring your calorie intake was hard, I'm going to tell you that that was the easy part. The truly impossible task is to measure your energy output. Until we figure out a way to install an energy gauge that's screwed into the middle of your forehead that will measure how many calories you are burning per minute, you won't know the answer. There are books that have the gall to say that you burn up so many calories per minute sitting in a chair or playing tennis or walking or doing any one of hundreds of other activities. I challenge anyone who has produced one of these tables to prove that they are anything more than wild guesses.

On a Sunday morning, when I go out to play tennis, there may be 30 or more people out there doing the same thing. I doubt that during any single hour any one of them will burn up exactly the same number of calories as any other one. They are different ages, sizes, and genders, and have differing degrees of skill and physical conditioning. It would not be surprising if some burn up three times as many calories per hour as others do. Yet they might each go to the same little book that they bought at the checkout counter and learn that they had each burned up the same number of calories per hour playing tennis.

There are a number of ways to attempt to actually measure how many calories a person burns up at a specific activity. One method involves putting that individual into a closed chamber and measuring the heat that he produces while performing some activity. Can you picture a chamber built just for tennis alone? It would have to be some sort of enormous bubble over the court. But then you would have to have two people in it. Tennis isn't played alone. What if you couldn't assume that heat production of each individual was identical? I'm being facetious. The idea is total nonsense.

You can also measure calorie consumption by allowing a person to breathe measured amounts of oxygen and observe the amount of carbon dioxide he exhales. This takes quite a bulky apparatus including tanks of oxygen. Even if you could strap all this to a tennis player, do you think you could count on his performance that day to be representative of one of his typical tennis outings without all that baggage?

Let's not go on with this. I maintain that you can't even come close to measuring a person's daily caloric expenditure. This is one of the few dogmatic statements I shall make in this whole book. I feel I'm on pretty firm ground with this one.

Then what good is it to try to balance your calorie intake with your calorie expenditure? The answer is that it has some value. In fact, I'm guilty of regularly making the attempt. It's better than not trying.

So why have I gone to the trouble of telling you all this? I don't want you to believe everything you read or hear. Skepticism is good. Doubt helps us survive. You're going to pick up a newspaper one day and read that Dr. Siegal's diet ideas are too radical. The article will be written by some authority who has never stopped to question The Great Calorie Theory, someone who believes that he knows how many calories he eats every day and how many he burns up, someone whose experience with actual overweight people is nil. He may have gotten A's in nutrition school. That's his claim to fame.

Don't discount everything you read or hear about nutrition, just question it. Ask yourself, "How does the author know this? How did he come by this information? Is he repeating what he heard or what he read in someone else's article?

I apply The Great Calorie Theory in my approach to weight loss even though I know it's flawed. I may even spout it out to patients as though it were gospel. It serves the purpose. It enables me, in spite of its flaws, to help thousands of people take off weight. If you remember, I've said I'm a practical man. TGCT doesn't have to be perfect. If it helps in what I'm doing, I can settle for it even though I recognize its limitations—at least until something better comes along.

The moral of this story: don't automatically believe everything you read or hear.

# Chapter 13

# The Last Ten Pounds
# Are the Hardest

The chapter title represents a common belief among those who have ever attempted to lose weight. They are correct, but I'll bet that very few have ever taken the time to analyze why that is so. There must be some plausible explanation for it. Let's see if we can get some clues.

Are you a body builder? If not, let's pretend that you are. So now, body builder, let's suppose you have just entered the gym and are doing your usual things with the weights for an hour. Is there any question that when you've finished, you've burned up some extra calories? By extra, I mean you've burned more calories than you would have burned if you hadn't been at the gym but rather had pursued your normal daily activities during that hour.

Of course, lifting those weights burns up some calories. It's argued that you might have burned more with an hour of aerobic activity, but we're not comparing exercise systems here. It's enough that you realize that you burn up some extra calories while pumping iron. Now suppose your hour at the gym were spent less productively. All you did was pick up a 25 pound weight and carry it around with you as you walked around the gym or socialized with the other folks for that hour. Clearly, you would have burned more calories than you would have without that 25 pounder. We don't know how many. In fact, I defy anyone to tell me how we could possibly accurately measure how many calories (even though some claim they can). It's enough that we accept that you would have burned up extra calories by carrying that weight.

Now let's suppose that when you left the gym, you did not leave the 25 pound weight behind. Instead you carried it with you, and as a matter of fact, you never put it down until you went to bed that night. You performed all your usual daily tasks while carrying that extra weight. Do you think you would have burned up more calories that day than you would have on a similar day without the extra weight? Isn't the answer obvious?

Now let's forget about that 25 pound weight and make a different supposition. Suppose you were 25 pounds heavier than you currently are. Would you not expect to burn up the same number of calories in a day as you would carrying the 25 pound weight in your hands? What difference does it make if you carry the weight in your hands or if it's strapped to your middle (beneath your skin as a big glob of fat) as you do your chores?

The answer is that there is no difference. Carrying 25 extra pounds is the same whether it's some external weight or part of your body. It takes extra effort to carry it in both cases, and that burns calories.

You will burn more calories as a result of your extra weight than if you were thinner. But here's the catch: that's true only if your activity level remains the same with those extra pounds.

In my medical practice, I see people who come to me with an extra 25 pounds. These are the exception. More often than not, they have 50 extra pounds. And quite a few have 100 or more. And there are even some in the 200-plus range of extra weight.

Can you imagine how many extra calories a day these folks are burning just to keep up with their *usual* activities? Pay some attention to that word, *usual*. As the weight increases, it becomes more difficult to maintain your usual activities, yet I'm amazed at how many seem to do just that. I'm reminded of a 500 pound patient who swore to me he had an active job that required him to be on his feet all day. I can't even begin to guess how many calories he used just to be able to walk around all day.

Elsewhere in the book, we've talked about caloric maintenance levels. To clarify, that's the average number of calories you burn per day performing your usual activities. It should now be clear to you that for every pound you gain, you also increase your burning of calories a little bit, so in a sense, your own weight helps you to keep it in check. Your own weight helps you to take it off!

Although a noted professor of exercise physiology has published data to suggest that the number of calories we burn for a specific activity (even sedentary) is directly proportional to body weight, I'm not convinced that there is such an absolutely direct relationship. My own experience with my patients clearly indicates that the heavier the patient, the more calories burned per hour. Yet I have trouble accepting that a 200 pound lady burns twice the calories of a 100 pound counterpart with the exact same physical activity.

Let's play it safe and leave it at *the heavier you are, the more calories you burn for the same activity.*

Of course, keeping your regular activity level becomes more difficult as you gain weight. That means that the benefit of the extra calorie burning is offset somewhat by the slowing down of your activities. Eventually, as you gain, the two should reach equilibrium. As your excess weight contributes to calorie burning, your reduced activity lessens it. Finally, the reduced activity takes over and the excess weight is not nearly as helpful in reducing itself.

In Chapter 21, I ask you to take the step of measuring your caloric maintenance level as a prelude to starting your diet. You can then make various other calculations based on your objectives. Do you want to reach a certain goal weight by some specific date? Or do you want to know when you can expect to reach your goal weight based on how many calories you eat per day? All of these results will depend on your Daily Caloric Maintenance Level. If you check the Web site CookieDiet.com, you can access a test called Dr. Siegal's 28-Day Calorie Burn Rate Self-Test that will enable you to get all that information.

If you have a lot of weight to lose, that Daily Caloric Maintenance Level should decrease as you lose weight. You should, from time to time, freely recheck it by repeating the test. It should be repeated at least after each 25 pounds you lose. That won't be difficult because your diet is itself the test. The added burden is jotting down some numbers.

It isn't exactly the last 10 pounds that are more difficult but rather that during the entire weight-loss effort, as the pounds come off and you no longer have to drag them around with you, you don't burn those extras calories needed to carry them.

How can you compensate for this slowing of your progress as you near your goal? That's easy—well maybe not that easy. By increasing your physical activity consistent with your weight loss you tend to nullify this process. Or, you could regularly strap on to your body extra pounds of weight equal to what you had lost. Sounds like it would work, but it's highly impractical. People might talk.

So there you have it. I hope I've given you an understanding of what's involved in one aspect of weight loss, something that I doubt you've ever seen in a diet book before. This is good information. Use it to your advantage. Don't let the gradual slowing discourage your effort. It's the best evidence that you're accomplishing something.

# Chapter 14

# But Doctor, I Don't Overeat

Would it surprise you to hear that many patients have complaints about their doctors? I didn't think it would. Quite often it's a patient's "last" doctor. That's another way of saying that he is no longer her doctor. Some complaints are very generic: they might apply to any physician, regardless of specialty. "I have to wait forever." "He's very aloof." "She never returns my calls." Other complaints relate directly to questioning the doctor's ability in his specialty.

That's the kind I hear most. Since my own specialty is treating overweight people, for some reason, I seem to hear more than the usual amount of doctor complaints. And those I hear are remarkably similar. I'll give you to the end of this sentence to guess the nature of this common complaint. Time's up. My patients tell me that their former doctors believed that they were lying to them. What's more, they were all accused of the same lie. Of course, it wasn't necessarily an overt accusation. It was usually more subtle, more diplomatic, more like this. "That's probably not exactly the case," or "It's easy to misjudge." The doctor, relying on his experience with lots of patients, couldn't believe that their assertions were true.

The lie? "I don't overeat."

About 25 percent of my new patients truly don't overeat and yet are overweight.

Here's an invented dialogue that will lay it out for you.

> *Former doctor:* Clearly, your problem is your weight. You've got to start eating sensibly.
>
> *Patient:* But, Doctor, I do eat sensibly.
>
> *Former doctor:* No, I mean that you've got to stop overeating.
>
> *Patient:* I don't overeat. I'm very careful. I just can't lose weight.
>
> *Former doctor:* Hmm. I see.
>
> *Patient:* Doctor, I know there's something wrong with my metabolism. I eat like a bird. Everyone around me eats twice as much, and they're all thin.
>
> *Former doctor:* Do you remember those tests we did two weeks ago? They showed that your metabolism is normal. We tested your thyroid. Normal. There's nothing wrong with your metabolism. Let's start pushing away from the table.

Sure, I invented this dialogue, but I swear I've had many patients report conversations with their doctors that were virtually identical.

So what's going on? The patient says she eats like a bird, and the doctor says (or, at least implies), "You're lying."

Of course the doctor knows that there are some people who, although quite overweight, don't overeat. In other words, given the quantity that they eat, they shouldn't have gained weight. The doctor also knows that this happens frequently in people who have hypothyroidism. He knows who has hypothyroidism because he knows the symptoms and he knows that the laboratory tests that he does will confirm it. He can trust the laboratory to make the diagnosis.

Or can he? To borrow from Gershwin, "It ain't necessarily so."

Here's the point. Medical laboratories are wonderful. The hundreds of tests that they do are invaluable to the physician. They contribute heavily to saving lives. The tests don't make the diagnosis, but they sure help the doctor to do just that. But as good as they may be, the tests aren't always accurate. We can argue forever as to whether such errors are excusable, but I don't care to get into that. I'm not complaining about the errors.

What I'm questioning is the actual value of some specific tests. I rely on the results of laboratory tests constantly in my practice. But I do not trust all of them. Most doctors have their own biases when it comes to the value of specific tests. I'm in that category. But I'm certainly in the minority when it comes to the value of tests that relate to the function of the thyroid gland.

So before we go any further, let's take a look at the thyroid and what it does. You don't need to know an awful lot about the gland itself, but here are a few facts. The thyroid gland is located at the base of the neck, right below the Adam's apple. It manufactures chemicals that it dumps right into the bloodstream. These are the hormones that regulate metabolism or, more simply, how one turns fat into energy (the kind of energy that scientists speak about, not the bouncy behavior of "energetic" persons). Our subject today is not getting enough of these hormones.

It is universally accepted that if you eat more calories in a day than you need to run your body that day, you store those extra calories as fat. You gain a little weight. It seems that the thyroid gland is what influences how many calories you need to run your body by regulating the rate at which you "burn" calories. We might call this rate your metabolic rate. As we have said, the thyroid secretes hormones that are the substances that regulate this fat burning. If the supply of hormones is inadequate, the rate of burning calories may be diminished. Translation: If your thyroid gland doesn't produce, you gain unexpected weight. By the same token, if you're dieting, you may not lose as fast as expected.

These thyroid hormones are released into the bloodstream by the thyroid gland when needed and when everything is working properly. But as you may have discovered, things don't always work properly.

When there is an inadequate supply of hormones from the thyroid gland, the resulting condition is hypothyroidism, an often misdiagnosed condition, the symptoms of which include difficulty losing weight. Too *much* thyroid hormone results in the opposite condition, hyperthyroidism, which does not generally make you fat and, therefore, is not a subject of this book. Nonetheless, you should know that in those who suffer from *hyper*thyroidism, the disease is often converted to *hypo*-thyroidism by none other than the doctors who treat it. This is not an exposé of bad doctors. The unintended conversion from one condition to the other is, unfortunately, the result of good treatment. It is the expected result of surgery or other techniques for either partially removing the thyroid gland or inactivating it. Thus, the former hyperthyroidism sufferer now has hypothyroidism.

As if making you fat is not enough, hypothyroidism is responsible for more inconvenient symptoms than I can shake a fist at. Here is a list of 24 of them, and it's probably not complete:

Anemia
Brittle nails
Cold intolerance
Constipation
Depression
Dry or coarse hair

Dry skin
Fatigue
Hair loss
Headaches
Hoarse voice
Impotence
Infertility
Irritability
Low body temperature
Memory loss
Menstrual pain and other abnormalities
Miscarriages
Muscle pain and cramps
Palpitations
Puffy facial features
Sleeping excessively
Slow pulse
Weakness

Now you can see how easy my job is. All I have to do is to examine and question my patient, and if she has all of these 24 symptoms and is also overweight, she has hypothyroidism. That's easy. Not so fast! This particular ailment is both devious and perverse. You see, I've never seen anyone with hypothyroidism who had all of the symptoms. Hypothyroidism likes to dole out a few to one person and another random group of them to the next victim. Men particularly always miss some of them. (That was a joke!)

There is sort of an unwritten law in medicine: if something is missing, supply it. I'm not going to go into examples; they should be obvious. And that's how doctors treat hypothyroidism. They supply what's missing: thyroid hormone. For the record, there are two general types of thyroid hormone: the real stuff and the synthetic variety. Also for the record, the synthetic is easily 10 times as popular with doctors. I prefer the real type, which I call "natural" thyroid hormone. I could write volumes about this and, in fact, I did write one volume.[1]

I would like to say a word about natural thyroid hormone. What makes it real is that it's actually taken from the thyroid glands of cattle. When I began my medical practice many moons ago, that's all there was. It worked well. Shortly afterward, smart people figured out a way to make synthetic thyroid, which they said worked better. I don't think it does. I'm not alone in this belief, but I'm certainly in the minority.

At any rate, thyroid hormone is unquestionably the way hypothyroidism is treated. Both forms of the hormone are available in pill form. Every doctor knows this. Both types of thyroid hormone work, but there is some disagreement as to which works best.

So what do I mean by "It works"? Supplying thyroid hormone in the form of tablets manages hypothyroidism, or at least it relieves the symptoms. After diagnosing hypothyroidism in myriad patients, I can't begin to tell you for how many of those people symptoms disappeared. For the first time in years, headaches disappeared, depression was alleviated, and women became pregnant when they thought it could never happen.

Here is a word about psychological effects. The change in the personalities of patients once their hypothyroidism is properly treated may be more dramatic and noteworthy than their massive weight loss. I've seen dull, uncommunicative couch potatoes become absolute dynamos, extroverts. These were remarkable transformations.

All of this was fortuitous. None of these people came to me so I might eradicate their hypothyroid symptoms; they came to lose weight. As it happened, they not only lost the weight but also the misery of hypothyroidism.

In case I have failed to make my point, I'll condense it into the following paragraph:

---

[1] *Is Your Thyroid Making You Fat?* (Warner Books, 2000)

*There is a condition called hypothyroidism that affects about one out of four overweight individuals. It is at least partially responsible for their inability to achieve a normal weight. It is accompanied by a bunch of symptoms that seem totally unrelated to weight, some of which are more troublesome to the victim than the weight. The condition is routinely undiscovered by physicians who rely totally on the laboratory to make the diagnosis, and the laboratory does an inadequate job of doing so. As a result, the doctor believes his patient is overweight because of a lack of discipline or motivation. In short, he believes his patient, in reporting her eating habits, is fibbing. The hypothyroidism continues to take its toll. The patient's weight does not improve. A variety of symptoms continues. The patient is unhappy with the doctor because he doesn't believe her. That's the end of the story unless the patient takes the bull by the horns and invokes self-help.*

Don't take this as a mandate to automatically mistrust your doctor. What I have condensed into the preceding paragraph certainly does not apply to all doctors and definitely not to any doctor's ability to diagnose disease. I consider this to be an isolated aberration of the usual doctor-patient relationship. It probably stems from three factors. The first is too much confidence in anything that hides under the mantle of high-tech science. "Who am I to question those expensive machines?"

The second is that any experienced physician expects patients to lie. Part of the art of medicine is the ability to evaluate the truthfulness of the information given you by the patient. Author Ernest Hemingway prided himself in having a "built-in...shit detector." Not all doctors have one.

The third and perhaps most important is the almost universal belief among doctors, as well as everyone else, that being overweight is a character flaw and that it is always due to just eating too much. In fact, it *is* due to eating too much. But "too much" for someone with hypothyroidism might not be very much. That amount might be just the right amount for someone without hypothyroidism.

So how can you reconcile your doctor's dismissal of your opinion that your metabolism may not be normal? You need to give him a little more help than usually accompanies the typical doctor-patient relationship. It's worth a try.

Try something such as this. You might say that you read a book by this crackpot, Dr. Siegal, in which he suggests that sometimes hypothyroidism is missed even though the laboratory denies it. Dr. Siegal has, on his Web site, a test to evaluate the rate at which you burn calories (see Chapter 21).

> *"On the CookieDiet.com Web site, Dr. Siegal has this test that's easy to do, and I did it. I ate exactly 1,000 calories a day for 28 straight days. I weighed myself very carefully at the beginning and the end. I lost weight but only two pounds. His test indicated that my daily caloric maintenance level was only 1,250 calories. Isn't that very low?"*

You'd better leave it at that, but you could add one more thing. You might include, "Can *you* think of any reason for this other than hypothyroidism?"

I can't advise you beyond this. The ball is now in the doctor's court. He has a choice: he can believe you about your test or not. If he questions your honesty, what can I say? If he believes you, I can't imagine what kind of alternative explanation he can come up with. I can tell you, I've talked to a lot of doctors about this over the years, and there are those who not only understand the concept completely, but who've actually observed the same phenomenon in their own patients.

And if this approach fails, what then? You might want to get a second opinion.

The bottom line is if you think you have a metabolic problem, and that is to say, you truly eat reasonably and are still overweight, take action. Test yourself as I have suggested in Chapter 21. Present the results to your doctor (or some doctor). If you are lucky enough to form a relationship with a doctor who is willing to go beyond the stereotypes that are assigned to the overweight population, it can change your life. It's worth the effort. But remember, hypothyroidism exists in only one out of four overweight individuals. The odds are still in favor of overeating as the cause of your problem.

# Chapter 15

# Faster Is Better

Alot of people who don't know what they're talking about
will tell you that losing weight gradually is better than
losing it quickly. Well, they're just plain wrong. Worse,
whatever explanation they offer (if they even bother since usually
the explanation is simply "because it is") is based on something they
heard or read, not on the experience of a real person. Whereas, as
noted in Chapter 2, my opinions are based largely on my experience treating more than a half million overweight patients and,
therefore, constitute anecdotal evidence, those opinions of the
"you shouldn't lose too fast" faction can best be characterized as
urban myth.

Of course, there is absolutely no consensus among those who
espouse such nonsense as to what is meant by *gradual* or how
quick is *too* quick. I've heard nutritionists, people on the health
professions fringe, and even my fellow physicians say that anywhere
from two to five pounds per month is the "right" rate and that 10
or more a month (the rate I shoot for) is dangerous.

Again, while claiming that rapid weight loss is dangerous, its
opponents never produce an actual harmed person to support their

positions. By contrast, I have referred to the media many of my patients as well as CookieDiet.com customers who've lost a lot of weight fast. Their stories have been told by ABC's *Good Morning America*, NBC's *The Today Show*, *The Fox Morning Show*, *Forbes*, *It's Your Call with Lynn Doyle*, *Entertainment Tonight*, and other major media outlets. Did you see the cover of the January 12, 2009 *People* magazine? It featured a photograph of Josie Raper, a young woman from Phoenix who actually lost half her body weight on Dr. Siegal's Cookie Diet.

## Hunger Control and a Motivated Dieter: Keys to Successful Weight Loss

Dr. Siegal's Cookie Diet is rooted in two observations that I first made shortly after I began practicing medicine in 1957: (1) hunger wrecks diets and (2) the faster the weight comes off, the more likely the dieter is to reach her goal.

In this book, I've covered extensively the first one, that hunger control is a requirement for diet success. Equally important is the motivation of the dieter. Is there any question that this is true? Think about your own experiences. Is there anything more motivating than getting on the scale and seeing that you've dropped another three pounds this week? Conversely, how have you felt when you've discovered that for your week's worth of discipline and sacrifice your reward was a measly pound or so? Did you say to yourself, "Whoopee, another pound! Just another eight months of deprivation to go!"? More likely, it was something like, "At this rate I'll never get there anyway. Pass the potatoes, please."

A diet consisting of 1,000 calories a day is safe when your doctor determines that your medical history and condition warrant such a regimen and that he or she monitors your health as you diet. The laws of human physiology (and my half century of experience) indicate that most people lose about 10 pounds per month on a

1,000 calorie diet. Therefore, I reiterate: a 1,000 calorie diet safely results in rapid weight loss.

## If You Suspend Your Diet Before You Reach Your Goal, You Won't Resume It Until You've Gained Back Much of the Weight You Had Lost.

A realization that's been reinforced countless times in my career is that if my patient "falls off the wagon" before reaching her goal, she's unlikely to resume her diet where she left off. In other words, she won't maintain the weight she had when she prematurely ended her diet. Before she's again motivated to attempt to lose weight, she'll first regain much of the weight she had lost. I can only speculate as to the reason for this phenomenon. My belief is that nearly all of us have an upper weight threshold, a level of dissatisfaction that we must reach before we'll take corrective action. Possibly, we gradually add pounds until one day we say to ourselves, "Enough." The trigger can be almost anything, such as the sight of oneself in a bathing suit; setting a new record on the scale; or for us men, looking down in the shower and not seeing a familiar friend.

Viewed on a continuum, the variations in those thresholds are extreme. At either end are those who may have no threshold at all. They are the anorexics, whose upper thresholds may be fatally low, and the morbidly obese, who can reach 1,000 pounds or more and die before ever resolving to put a stop to the madness.

Here's how it often comes about. You begin a diet at 225 pounds and your goal is 160 pounds. If you interrupt your diet at 195 pounds, it's likely that you won't be motivated to resume it until you're back to the point that prompted you to start the diet in the first place. It makes sense if you think about it. At your current weight of 195 pounds, you look and feel a lot better than you did so recently at 225 pounds. It's easy to get complacent at this point and think that your current level is "good enough" and that you "deserve" the time off. Please heed my advice and avoid that trap. Once you start your diet, see it through to the end.

So why do some people stop before they reach their goals? For some, it's probably subconsciously intended; they stop because they're afraid to go on. There is no question that I've had plenty of patients who clearly wanted—even needed—to fail. I'm not a psychiatrist, and yet a few patients have confessed to me that, as the weight began to come off, their anxiety level increased. The world treats overweight people differently, and going from very overweight to thin often presents opportunities (especially social and professional ones) that so recently were unavailable. That can be frightening for some. One's excess weight often serves as a convenient excuse or explanation for one's lack of success in some area. To reduce the weight is to weaken the excuse. If the weight can no longer be blamed, one must now face the real cause of one's failure.

For most people, however, I'm convinced that they stop because their progress is too slow to sustain their motivation. A lot of patients have come to me over the years while on Weight Watchers, a program that absolutely results in weight loss but does so at a modest pace. Like any plan that produces a caloric deficit, Weight Watchers works if you follow it and stay with it. In my experience, however, in this age of fast food, instant communications, and "real time" everything, most people are impatient. They don't want fast; they want faster. They want fastest.

Dr. Siegal's Cookie Diet, when scrupulously followed according to all of the instructions in this book, safely results in the fastest possible weight loss, and contrary to what you may have heard, fast weight loss fosters success.

# Chapter 16

# Scientific Research

We are barraged with information on nutrition. It bombards us from all directions: newspapers, radio, television, magazines, and of course, the Internet. What are we to believe? Common sense tells us that what we see and hear on the subject of nutrition (and, in fact, any other subject) can't all be trusted. It's obvious. Aren't we supplied with information that directly conflicts with other information?

If you are to be an intelligent and sophisticated receptacle for information beamed in your direction, you must train yourself to analyze carefully the words that comprise this information.

In the scientific literature and in the popular reporting of the results of experiments, a statement is frequently made that this or that has been shown to be associated with some other this or that. The operative phrase here is *associated with*, and it is important to understand the implications of this phrase.

Suppose some researcher had completed a study of the life expectancy of people from various economic groups. Assume that the study had shown that the individuals with highest incomes also had the longest life expectancy. At the low end of scale, the differences in life expectancy were even more dramatic. It showed that individuals at the poverty level were expected to have disproportionately shorter lives.

No one would be particularly surprised at these results. It is the kind of thing that we would expect. The researcher may have concluded his paper by stating that increased income is definitely associated with increased life expectancy.

Now let us suppose that he had gone one step further. Suppose that he had attempted to make this information more useful to the readers by giving them some fatherly advice. He might have added, "If you want to live to a ripe old age, be sure to make a lot of money."

Just how valid would this statement have been? The experiment certainly showed that having more money was *associated* with longer life, but was it the *cause* of the longer life? Quite obviously it was not the direct cause. Having money does not automatically prolong your stay on this planet. Something more has to take place to improve your life expectancy.

He might have done further experiments to show why there was an association between income and mortality. It might have shown that the affluent have the opportunity to eat a more healthful diet, to have the leisure time to exercise, or have access to better healthcare. Or it might indicate that the disadvantaged are exposed to more dangerous environments. It is ridiculous to think that all you have to do is win a lottery and your longevity is assured. It takes more than that. You have to do things with that money that will foster longevity. An example might be your buying a safer though more expensive car or perhaps moving out of a dangerous inner city to a costlier but safer suburb. Statistically, factors such as these could demonstrate why the wealthier might have a longer life expectancy.

We cannot deny that his experiment does show the relationship between wealth and prolonged life. But "associated with" does not necessarily imply "caused by."

Too often we make the assumption that because two events are associated, one is caused by the other. Sometimes we are led in this direction by others. The charge has been made that this has been done in reporting on the cholesterol question.

We might want to raise the question as to whether deaths from coronary heart disease are really caused by increased cholesterol in the blood. We might accept the fact that there is an association but not necessarily a causal relationship. For example, what if there were some other common factor frequently present in people with high cholesterol and it was this factor that caused the heart attacks? Perhaps it could be shown that those who had this factor in their lives frequently had heart attacks whether they had high cholesterol or not.

Suppose that factor was sugar. Remember, we are speculating here. I'm not saying it *is* sugar. I'm just trying to get you to fantasize and see what develops. Suppose someone did a study that showed that people who eat a lot of saturated fat in their diets generally are those who also eat a lot of sweets. That wouldn't be so surprising. But more experimentation would have to be done. We would need to know which of the two associated factors could really be the cause of heart problems. In the end we might find out that neither was the cause, but rather some other factor that was associated with sugar, fat, and blood cholesterol.

It may quite well be that there has not been sufficient research to warrant the extreme warnings that are given us as to fats in our diets. Yet who can dispute that prudence is wise? If there is even suspicion that fats are dangerous, should we not play it safe and avoid them? The answer seems simple enough. But this simple answer could be complicated if there were also some suspicion that the diminishment of fat intake itself might be harmful. Certainly the question has been raised that the so-called safe fats, the polyunsaturated fats, might not be all that safe.

What is needed is, of course, is the definitive experiment, the one that will tell us once and for all whether we should be eating fats or cholesterol or saturated fats or unsaturated fats or . . .

That seems easy enough. If we are going to blame the research community for dragging their collective feet in not supplying us with the information we need to enjoy a happy and long life, let us take the bull by the horns and solve this problem ourselves. Let's go through a little exercise here. Let's take that first step and design that experiment.

What is it that we want to know? In terms of the information given in this book, we would like to know whether eating a diet high in saturated fat or the current villain, trans fat, results in a population that dies earlier than another population that eats the current "prudent" diet.

We are going to need two groups of human subjects. One of these groups, Test Group A, will be fed a diet high in saturated (animal) fat. The other group, Test Group B, will be fed a diet of only moderate fat, and these fats will be made up principally of polyunsaturated oils such as safflower and monounsaturated oils such as olive.

But wait a minute. Hasn't this already been done? Haven't large population groups been studied in terms of their diets over a period of years? Yes, they have. We don't have to repeat those studies. But can we rely on the tests that have been done? Maybe we can't.

I have been asking questions regarding the daily diets of my own patients for many years. It is sometimes very trying. Quite often I am aware that I am not getting honest answers. Dishonest answers are not always intentionally dishonest. They are simply part of some psychological machinations that go on inside our heads. Too often patients tell me about the diet they would *like to think* they've been eating.

I would like to have a nickel for every time I've had a conversation with a patient that went something like this:

*Dr. S:* Do you believe that you overeat?

*Patient:* Absolutely not. My husband eats three times as much as I do.

*Dr. S:* Do you eat between meals?

*Patient:* Not usually, although I do like to have a snack late in the afternoon.

*Dr. S:* What do you have then?

*Patient:* I'm at work then. I might have a bag of potato chips or a candy bar and maybe a can of soda.

*Dr. S:* But you don't do that in between breakfast and lunch?

*Patient:* Well, I may have a doughnut or something during my morning coffee break.

*Dr. S:* What about after dinner?

*Patient:* No. But I may have some ice cream or something before I go to bed.

*Dr. S:* What about your meals?

*Patient:* Dinner is our big meal, although sometimes I go overboard with lunch.

*Dr. S:* Do you eat much breakfast?

*Patient:* That's the one meal I really need. I can't function without a good breakfast.

*Dr. S:* Don't you feel that the three meals plus all the in-between eating might be more than you need?

*Patient:* I guess that it is. But, you know, I don't really eat very much. Like today. I was in a hurry to make this appointment. I had hardly any lunch.

I hope you see the point. It's so difficult to get an accurate history from a patient. They are inconsistent. They lie to themselves, and they lie to me. And they don't even know that they're lying. In one breath they confess to being gluttons and immediately follow with a description of their Spartan diets.

Researchers unfortunately face the same problems in questioning their subjects. They get their information from face-to-face interviewers who may be students working part time in that capacity to supplement their incomes. They themselves may be poorly motivated to do a good job. Worse, the research subjects may do their reporting by answering written questionnaires. I'm not sure that the information that goes into our cholesterol studies or any other nutritional studies is very reliable. Remember, no one follows the subjects around constantly to observe what they really eat.

There is no question that my patients like to tell me what they think I want to hear. They're very kind. They don't want me to be disappointed. I would like another nickel for each time I was told that the patient across the desk had spent an entire month on virtually a total fast and, in the process, gained 10 pounds.

If we're to have a valid experiment, the information about our subjects' diets must be reliable. The only way to be absolutely certain that we're getting that kind of accurate information is to closely monitor all the meals and food that our subjects are eating. How can we do this? The answer is by having our subjects in a closed environment where all their activities are scrutinized. They will have to live in a facility where all their food is provided and where there is no possibility of cheating. They'll have to be watched 24 hours a day. After all, we don't want anyone sneaking unapproved food to them.

How many subjects will we need for our experiment? Remember, we're studying the effects of diet on mortality. Will 20 in each group be enough? I doubt it. At the end of our experiment, all 40 might still be alive and we will have proved nothing. I don't think we can get much useful information with groups of less than 1,000. Even that isn't very large. Of course, the larger the group, the more reliable the conclusions.

So for our experiment we are going to need at least 2,000 individuals who will essentially be captives, eat the foods we provide them, and allow us to study them over a period of time. Each time one dies, we will do an autopsy and determine the cause of death. We will, of course, tabulate the deaths from heart attacks in both groups. At the end of the experiment, we might be able to calculate through statistical techniques whether a saturated fat diet will kill you.

When will the experiment end? Should we run it for a month? Two months? Six months? No, this kind of study takes years.

No one would expect the results of these diets to be evident over short periods of time. The harmful effects of diet are generally the result of long-term changes. Experiments such as this need 20, 30, 40, or even more years. I don't know how old you are, but I can't realistically expect to be around at the conclusion of our experiment.

If you don't see the point yet, I'll give it to you straight. This experiment is impossible to perform. In our society you simply can't make prisoners of a few thousand people for a lifetime. It is frowned upon. The only ones in history that could have even contemplated such a study would have been the Third Reich, but fortunately the Nazis didn't last long enough.

The nature of these kinds of investigations makes them very difficult to accomplish. It requires the right subjects, the right controls over their lives, and sufficient time to see the results. The research institutions are not to be blamed for not doing the right experiments. This is not an easy subject to study. We have to do the best we can with what we can practically accomplish.

In my opinion, if there is any fault, it's in reading too much into the results of the research that's already been done. We are led to believe that the information regarding fats in the diet, blood cholesterol, and related subjects is gospel. Remember that proving an association between diet or blood constituents and heart attacks doesn't necessarily prove a causal relationship. It has even been suggested that there are vested interests that profit from slanted information given to us. If the justification for the current dietary recommendations is that we will be "playing it safe," we deserve to know the whole story so we can decide whether we want to play it safe.

So what about this 80-year-old guy who is telling you that he has administered a half million or so overweight people and has decided he knows a sure method to get your weight down and, thus, prolong your life or at least improve its quality? What are the chances that it's all a big lie? What are the chances that he's totally sincere and above board? You might bump into some of my patients—there are quite a few running around out there—and question them. Or you can read this entire book—I hope you will—and try to read between the lines and make your best guess. Or you can decide that anything that sounds this good can't be true. Or you can simply accept it on faith.

It's particularly hard for me to guide you since you've already sensed what a skeptic and cynic I've become after all these years. I want you also to be skeptical and cynical. It's a great defense against what's out there.

You should assess in your own mind the benefit of following my lead as compared to the risk involved in doing so. You do have something to lose—your weight.

Here goes that admonition again. If you're going to do it, do it with your doctor's help. I don't think he'll steer you wrong.

If the subject of scientific research has piqued your interest and you want to know more, move on to the next chapter for much more on the same general subject.

If, however, your eyes have already glazed over and in between yawns you're wondering if I'm ever going to tell you how to get thin, you have my permission to skip the next chapter. I'll understand.

## Chapter 17

# Scientific Integrity

Has this ever happened to you? You've heard or read something about a new scientific breakthrough that seemed to be terribly important and you waited to hear more about this marvel. Perhaps it was an item in the daily newspaper or on the television news.

You were told that scientists had discovered a promising treatment for some horrible disease or a new drug that could slow down aging or grow hair or make you more sexy. You made a mental note to learn more about it, but as the days passed, you were very busy and forgot all about the announcement. Then it came back to you, and you realized that you had never heard anything more about the miraculous discovery. What happened? This had been heralded as a momentous development. Why wasn't the media following up on this important story?

True scientific breakthroughs are quite rare. But there are a lot of suggestions of such groundbreaking discoveries. They reach us via the media. On a slow news day, these items are often used as "filler." But where do they come from? Are they mere inventions of some desperate reporter?

To understand the origins of articles whose titles are often, "New Hope for _____," you must understand a bit about scientific research and how the results of this research are reported to the world.

For example, let us suppose that some doctor who is employed by some organization that does research (a medical school, hospital, drug company, private research group, or government agency) has a suspicion that a certain known drug might have the effect of lowering blood cholesterol even though it has never been tried or tested for that purpose. Perhaps several doctors had reported that patients on this drug seemed to have lower cholesterol values than would be expected. One of the early tasks would be to design, on paper, an experiment that would test this concept. Good design for an experiment is terribly important. If the results are to be reliable, the design must be flawless.

Our research doctor would perhaps decide that he needs 50 subjects, all of whom have cholesterol readings between 200 and 350, on whom he will test this substance that he could give in the form of a pill. These subjects would be known as his *test group*. He will probably specify that he needs 50 more subjects who will serve as his *control group*. His experiment design specifies that he will give all of his subjects in both groups instructions as to the diet each will follow for the three months of the test. Both groups will follow the same diet. He will also instruct each of them that he or she must each day take the pill that is supplied. The pills given to the members of the test group will contain the substance he is testing. The other group, the control group, is to receive pills that look identical but that actually contain no drug. They are "sugar" pills, fakes, what doctors call "placebos." None of the subjects will know which group he is in, so he won't know if his pill is real or fake.

The researcher may or may not tell the subjects the purpose of the experiment, fearing that this might cause some individuals to alter their behavior to achieve a better result. For example, his instructions to them might be to eat their normal diet, but knowing that this is a cholesterol experiment could entice some subjects to eat fewer fats than usual to "help" the experiment. This would interfere with his goals. He would also have a duty to inform his subjects of any possible harm that could come to them as a result of following the instructions or of taking the pill. He would give the same instructions to all 100 even though 50 of them were taking the placebos.

All this could result in a delicate juggling act. He could be more confident of the results obtained if he could act as an absolute dictator and control every aspect of his subjects' behavior. If he had his choice, I'm certain he would prefer to be working with slaves or prisoners. His desire for a well-designed experiment is counterbalanced by his ethical and moral obligations to do the right thing with his subjects. He can't expose them to risks without their permission, and yet it is possible that the more they know, the more unreliable the results of the experiment will be.

What I have described is a great simplification of what actually occurs. In practice, it is much more complicated. He may not be able to start with humans at all. He may have to test his substance first on animals. Humans are problems. He wouldn't have to give his animal subjects complete disclosure. The rules don't require their "informed consent." That's one of the reasons animals are such popular subjects for research. However, he might have to deal with the animal rights people. The animal experiments themselves could occupy years of his time before he ever gets to try his pill on human subjects.

To make the results of his experiment even more valid, he might choose to keep himself ignorant of who is getting the real pill and who is getting the fake pill. This can be accomplished by allowing a computer to decide who gets the real pill and who gets the placebo. The computer keeps track of it, and after all the results are in, the computer reveals which subjects were in each group.

This kind of study, where even the experimenter is kept in the dark, is common and is called a "double-blind study." Its purpose is to ensure that the researcher will not unconsciously or accidentally slant the results of the experiment in one direction or another. Only when the testing phase is over and all the results are in and tabulated does he learn who took which pill.

He must include in the plan for his future experiment the schedule of how to monitor his subjects. Will he test their blood for cholesterol content periodically during the three months? When he reaches the end of the experimental period and does his final blood tests, how will he decide whether the pill was effective? What criteria will be used to evaluate success? All of these decisions and many more must be planned in advance to ensure that he will have scientifically valid conclusions that he and others can rely upon.

His experiment design might even include a second phase. In order to give his findings even more validity, at the conclusion of Phase One, just described, he could instruct all his subjects to go back to their normal pre-experiment lifestyle without the pills. Later he could again round them up and ask them to repeat the same experiment. However, this time he would give the real pills to the members of the previous control group and the fake pills to those who were formerly in the test group. By reversing the procedure, he would have sort of a double check on his results.

With plan in hand, he must now find someone to authorize his commencing with the experiment. The organization with which he is associated will probably have some kind of committee that evaluates proposals for experimental research and who will decide whether to authorize him to proceed. Someone will have to pay for this experiment. There will be salaries, materials, equipment, and innumerable other things that will cost money. These funds may come from his organization or they may have to go out and find a donor. The donor could be the government, which would be asked to give a grant to fund the experiment. It could be a private corporation that might stand to benefit if the results were to turn out in a certain way.

How does he get paid? Unless he is rich and donates his time, he has to live on his salary just like everyone else. He also would like his share of the luxuries of life. He could be a very ambitious person. He might be totally dedicated to science and yet still want as big a share of the pie as he can get.

He will make a salary, and this may come directly from those who fund the experiment. A government grant could include his salary, and it could even be a handsome salary.

Let us assume that the experiment design is submitted, it is approved, subjects are selected, the experiment is begun and finished, and the results are tabulated. There is a variety of conclusions possible. Suppose that in the group of 50 who actually took the test substance, the average blood cholesterol at the beginning of the experiment was 246, and the blood cholesterol average in the group that took the fake pills was 245. These two values would have been regarded as essentially identical. The baseline cholesterol reading for both groups was the same. If at the conclusion of the experiment, the test group had an average cholesterol of 209 and the control group had an average of 241, it could be concluded that taking the real pill had resulted in an impressive decrease in cholesterol values.

Of course, the honest researcher must be very careful that he is not ignoring some other factor that might have crept into the experiment. To have confidence in the results, every factor that the two groups were exposed to had to be identical with the exception that only one of the groups received the real drug.

Suppose the results had come out differently. What if the test group went from 246 to 239 and the control group average decreased from 245 to 243? Would this be significant? Could we say that the pill had some effect but not very much? Or could this change have been just the result of chance. The answer to this is complicated, and it is arrived at by some elaborate mathematical calculation that is beyond the scope of this book. There is a whole science devoted to analyzing experimental results and determining whether the results demonstrate some significant phenomenon. It is enough that you understand that results of experiments are not just black and white. They are often ambiguous and difficult to evaluate. Often even researchers will differ in their interpretations of the results of the same experiment.

Whether the experiment has proven that the pill lowers cholesterol or that it does not lower cholesterol could be equally important. Even a finding that the results were inconclusive could have some value in the future. Whatever the result, it should be reported so the scientific community has access to this information. It could save another researcher from spending money and wasting time in doing something that has already been done.

The conventional process by which experimental results are reported to the scientific community is publishing them in scientific journals. These journals are similar to magazines, generally published once a month, and are the storehouses of scientific information. They come in a variety of shapes, sizes, and formats. Like magazines, they have a number of articles, a table of contents, etc. Many carry no advertising. The articles are called "papers." A scientific paper is generally the complete description of an experiment, but it could also be a summation of the results of many experiments or the conclusions that a researcher has drawn from the combined experiments of others.

The usual destination for a scientific paper is the journal. An author may submit his paper to a number of journals before one accepts it for publication. Eventually, virtually everything gets published but not always in the most prestigious of journals. Very well-known journals with great stature include such publications as the *New England Journal of Medicine,* the *Journal of the American*

*Medical Association,* and *The Lancet.* There are many others that carry much prestige but are not as popular with the practicing physician, such as *Experimental Biology and Medicine.*

Scientific journals generally specialize; that is, they are devoted to a narrow field of science. Thus, a pediatric journal would probably not accept for publication those papers that deal with aging (geriatrics). Other journals are very broad in the scope of their interest. Some prestigious journals such as *Science* or *Nature* might choose to publish papers on very diverse subjects.

There are scientific journals for every imaginable branch of science. I concern myself mainly with those in the field of medicine, but sometimes fields overlap. Journals devoted to biology or chemistry could very well have a direct interest to someone in the medical field.

You will be impressed by how many journals exist. All the papers published in medical journals are catalogued. There is a master index of them that is constantly kept current. You could look up all the articles on the most narrow of subjects and actually read every paper ever written on that subject if you had the time. But you couldn't begin to subscribe to all these journals or to store them, so you would have to rely on special libraries as your source. It is also customary for each paper to make reference to many other papers, sometimes hundreds, and to clearly identify the exact journal, month, and page in which the referenced paper could be found. A physician trying to learn about a subject probably wouldn't have the time to do all that because the number of articles on even the narrowest of subjects is so vast that it would be impractical to attempt to digest them. One must, therefore, search out papers that attempt to summarize the available information. Textbooks essentially do this. They purportedly review all the information available and extract the meat from it. Needless to say, computers do a wonderful job of helping one to learn all about a subject.

More and more you will find books written by physicians and other medical professionals directed to the public rather than to the professionals. This book is such an example. Books of this type will often make reference to scientific papers and other sources but usually are much less technical than the papers published in journals. Of course, "diet books" have been around for a long time, but today a variety of subjects is covered by popular medical books. The old school in the medical hierarchy seems to frown on doctors communicating directly with the public through books, periodicals, or television. I've always felt that this was a type of elitism. Why should communication between a physician and the public be limited to his consultation room?

The master index for medical subjects published in journals up until 2004 was the Index Medicus. It was in the form of bound books and was in every library that specialized in medical subjects. Today it is replaced by electronic indexing in such amazing projects as MEDLINE or PubMed. Just try to fathom this. There are more than 5,000 journals that publish the results of medical experiments, and most of them come out each month. Each of these journals may contain as few as six papers or as many as 100. That means that every month, thousands of new medical papers are added to the storehouse of medical knowledge. This continues year after year. Each paper can occupy 50 pages or more in a journal. MEDLINE contains more than 18 million papers. If you were interested in a particular one of these papers, you might be able to read and understand it in 10 minutes, or you might spend months on a single paper and still not have a handle on its complete implications.

Obviously there is going to be duplication. Two or more groups may decide to research almost identical things. It may be intentional. Perhaps one will doubt the accuracy of what another paper reported and will repeat the experiment to see if they get the same results. It is conceivable that two groups may be investigating the same thing at the same time, not knowing that they are duplicating each other's efforts. This often happens when there is a lot of secrecy and there is actually a race to see who gets published first.

It is inevitable and sometimes disturbing that two similar experiments may be reported with vastly different results. It happens all the time. The authors and others will try to explain the reasons for the inconsistent results. The differences will often be explained by pointing out faulty experimental design on the part of the competition.

If the differences are the result of dishonesty, it could be very damaging to other researchers who might rely on the information that the paper supplied. Fraud in science is unfortunately real.

With this huge amount of information added each month, it is not difficult to find something contrary to even the most accepted of concepts. I have often felt that given enough time in the medical library, I could find some "scientific" substantiation for the most loony idea I could conceive.

By way of a far-out example, I (and other physicians) recognize that aspirin might be the wonder drug of the century. It is probably the most used drug of the past 100 years and is used for a variety of purposes. It relieves pain, lowers fever, and recently is a standard for preventing heart attacks and stroke. On the negative side, it has also been implicated in contributing to medical problems such as blood-clotting disorders and stomach ulcers. Although I have never done this, I would bet that I could research the studies that have been done on aspirin and offer some evidence that it could aid in the treatment or cure of many ailments for which it is not currently used. I could find as many papers that would say that aspirin is ineffective in treating those very same ailments. I could probably even find papers that say aspirin is effective in reducing cholesterol and other papers that offer proof that aspirin raises cholesterol. Of course, I'm only guessing about this to drive home my point. Don't hold me to it.

The amount of material is so immense that it is probable that you could find a paper that could be construed to support any idea you may have. This creates a field day for the media. They have an endless supply of material from which to draw. Let's invent a fictional newspaper, *The Podunk Herald*. If its staff wants to publish an article on a new drug for AIDS, they will have no trouble finding a paper that will substantiate that a drug was tested against the HIV virus. All they need is for an assistant to consult MEDLINE, and they will find all the ammunition they need. Their story could have been about an insignificant test done on animals with inconclusive results. The headline in *The Podunk Herald* might announce, "New Hope for AIDS Sufferers."

It is not surprising that many news stories deal with diet and drugs for weight loss. It's a hot subject. Do you now understand why you'll frequently read of a magical new drug for losing weight painlessly? I believe that at least several times a year for the past 50 or so, I have come across a story that suggests that the ultimate diet pill is just around the corner. Typically you read, "Researchers are studying the effects of a new drug that can be taken once a day and will allow you to eat all you want of fattening foods without gaining an ounce." Each time I read about one of these wonder drugs, it turns out to be an entirely new one. I have never read an article in the popular press that said, "The wonder drug we told you about last year turned out not to work" or "to be so dangerous that it could not possibly be released to the public."

What the media outlets don't ever seem to tell you is that later studies discredited the earlier study or that no further research was ever done on the subject because no one wanted to invest money in the lamebrain project.

So you read about this fantastic breakthrough and you never hear of it again. Is it a little clearer now why this happens?

If you are to become a sophisticated reader of *The Podunk Herald*, it will help if you understand where this medical information comes from and how it got into the newspaper. I'm not telling you to dismiss everything you read. I am telling you to evaluate everything, knowing the limitations of the system.

Can we rely upon anything we read? This is obviously a question that extends beyond what is written on scientific subjects. Most of us have no difficulty questioning what is written about world affairs or what is said by politicians. We have come to expect them to be devious and to be interested in furthering their own ends. We somehow endow our scientists and doctors, particularly those who do research, with virtues that no one possesses.

The perfect scientist would be one who single-mindedly cares about nothing except the search for truth. He would be completely objective. He would not be swayed by personal feelings and would not care in the least how his experiment turned out. One result would be as acceptable as its opposite. Truth would be all that matters. Furthermore, he would not be influenced in any way by personal gain, either financial or through notoriety or prestige. In short, he would be the perfect man, an ideal rather than a real live human being. Probably none of us possesses this combination of qualities. I believe that there are those out there who actually come close to this model, but I don't know who they are, and therefore, I don't know whom I can trust unequivocally.

More often these researchers are "just plain folks" like you and I, though perhaps a little smarter. They have the same or similar needs. They want to be recognized for the quality of their work. They want the satisfaction of having done some good things. They want to be compensated. They want to provide for their families and enjoy some of the good things in life. And therein lies the rub.

Can any researcher be truly objective? Can anyone who is testing to see if a drug to lower cholesterol is effective really not care whether it does or doesn't? If a particular researcher who is testing the drug happens to be paid by a grant from the government, and the result of his experiment shows that the drug has promise, might he not get another grant to study the subject in greater depth? Might this not guarantee his income into the future? Do these grants not support him, indeed provide him with luxuries? Can he truly be unbiased?

Obviously, one can be biased yet honest. A researcher can know that a particular result from his experiment may not be in his own best interests, yet his integrity will force him to be scrupulously honest and publish the information. But we are all driven by unconscious forces that color our actions. Even when dealing with a researcher with the most lofty of principles, there is still room to cast doubt on how objective the experiment really was.

Even if the researcher is a paragon of integrity, his benefactors might not be quite as pure. If a drug company is supplying his medical school with the funds to do his experiments, and his salary, his future, his prestige, and his whole life are tied up in the results of his experiments, is there not a little room to doubt his objectivity? This is not to suggest that they will pressure him to arrive at a particular conclusion, but would he not feel the pressure without any overt coercion from them?

Why am I telling you all of this? Why am I knocking myself out writing all these words? Am I really saying that I want you to disbelieve everything that you read in print? No, that's not it. If I were to tell you to disbelieve everything you read, my warning would necessarily have to include this very book.

Yet I do want you to leave room to doubt this book. It will be good exercise for your brain. You'll notice as you read this book that I seem to question many of my own past ideas. I believe that that is the way it should be. That is what I believe an intelligent and sophisticated observer or reader or consumer should do.

Question everything! Don't accept anything just because some "expert" says it is so, even if that expert is this author. Just because something appears in print does not make it so. Have more confidence in your own native intelligence and intuition.

Understand what motivates the people who do research and espouse their theories. Weigh carefully and, in the end, make your own decisions.

I smash some idols within these pages. I cast doubt on some of these sacrosanct principles of diet and nutrition. I don't ask you to participate in the smashing of these idols, but rather to consider carefully whether the contrary views have any merit. My own confidence in the popular standards of nutrition has been shaken by personal experiences over the years and how they differ from the reported experiences of a host of others. They have not made me a believer or a disbeliever, but rather, a skeptic.

Be a skeptic. But be an informed skeptic.

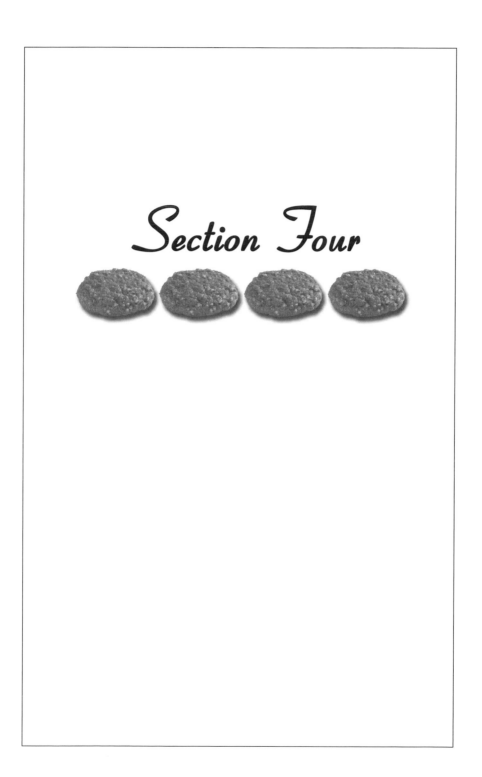

Section Four

## Chapter 18

# First, Consult Your Doctor

I say it a lot. I say it in media interviews. It's all over CookieDiet.com. I repeat it *ad nauseam* throughout this book. And I'll say it again now: do not go on a weight-loss diet— any weight-loss diet—except under the supervision of a qualified physician.

When I say that you should have your doctor monitor you, I don't necessarily mean that he should monitor your weight loss. He doesn't need to; on 1,000 (or even 1,200) calories, results are guaranteed. Humans simply cannot maintain their weight on so few calories.[1] What I mean is that he should evaluate your health, both *before and during* the weight-losing phase of your diet.

---

[1] If you're shaking you're head and saying, "That's not true, Dr. Siegal! I eat like a bird and can't lose weight," I've heard it a million times. While it's possible that you have a metabolic problem (see Chapter 14) that makes it harder for you than most others to lose weight, it's more likely that you're underestimating your caloric intake. It's very easy to do, and later in this book I give suggestions for more accurately measuring calorie consumption.

Why do I insist? There are several reasons, the most important of which is this: I want you to succeed. The last thing you need is another diet failure. The evidence is overwhelming that dieters are more successful when they are medically supervised. (Don't ask me to justify my position; my evidence is anecdotal.) Please note the following other reasons.

**A low-calorie diet might not be right for you.** First, your doctor should do a physical examination and lab work similar to what we do in my south Florida medical practice, Siegal Medical Group. This includes an EKG and bank of blood tests. He should determine if you are diabetic or are at risk for diabetes. He should evaluate your blood pressure and treat it if necessary. In short, your doctor must determine if it is safe for you to follow the diet. To make it easier for him to do so, you should bring him a copy of this book and ask him to read the chapter I wrote for him, Chapter 23, entitled "For Your Doctor's Eyes Only."

Once your doctor approves you to embark on a 1,000 calorie diet (or a modified version as he sees fit), his role has only just begun. You should return for checkups at whatever intervals he suggests.

Your doctor will look for adverse events. I don't expect there to be any, but it's always prudent to check for signs of trouble. I never see any serious problems from a low-calorie diet in my own patients. Occasionally a patient will complain of constipation, and I'll suggest using a laxative if the problem persists.

**People usually follow their doctor's instructions.** There is a natural tendency for patients to want to please their doctors. I see it in my own patients all the time. When a patient misses an appointment, it's usually because she has cheated on her diet and doesn't want to disappoint me. I doubt that this phenomenon is unique to the doctor-patient relationship. Surely it applies to teachers and students, fitness trainers and clients, and many other relationships where one party is an authority figure. Did you ever skip a class because you hadn't studied and didn't want the teacher to know?

I know I did. Losing weight is nobody's idea of fun even under the best of circumstances. If a desire to please (or not to disappoint) your doctor gives you even the slightest additional motivation to succeed, isn't it another good reason to see him?

And as if you need another reason, here it is. We are all vulnerable. We all in our lifetimes acquire anything from minor medical annoyances to serious illnesses. When dieting, it is human nature to assign blame for any symptom that occurs to the diet. Quite often it is unrelated, but the diet gets the blame. The result is that the patient stops the diet and loses what was destined to be a great benefit to her. Had her doctor clearly determined that whatever was bothering her was not related to the diet, she would not have stopped.

Are we clear on this? Please, see your doctor first.

## Chapter 19

# Nude Weighing
# in Public

I knew you'd read this chapter. Curiosity is powerful.

In brief, what you weigh during the course of your weight-losing effort is probably useful information, at least in contributing to your continued motivation. Because of the differences in the weights of your various items of clothing, it is desirable to know what you *actually* weight, that is, what you weigh while in your birthday suit.

Home scales, even costly ones, tend not only to be inaccurate, but worse, their accuracy can vary from day to day, particularly with temperature changes. Don't be fooled by the digital readouts. They're cute but probably no more accurate. If you have a "doctor's scale" with those sliding weights, you can count on it and won't have to get your nude weight in public places. If you don't have a really reliable scale, try to find a public one that looks substantial and use that same scale every time you weigh.

In my area of the country, the supermarket chain Publix has these great scales in every store and you don't have to put coins in them to make them work. They're free and look to be of very high quality. I've also seen good scales in other public places, even banks. It's time to assure you that if you follow my instructions for getting your nude weight, the odds are that you won't be embarrassed, that you won't attract a crowd, that you won't cause traffic jams, and what's most important, you won't spend the night in jail.

The secret is this: you need to know what your clothes weigh. And I'm not talking about just any clothes; I mean your "weighing clothes." You need to choose a particular outfit and designate it your *weighing clothes*. Pick out a complete outfit, every single item that you are willing to put on each time you weigh: underwear, shoes, everything. You are going to use these very same clothes every time you weigh.

The next step is to pack them all into a very light-weight plastic bag and cart them to a public scale that you will be using repeatedly in the future. You want to know the exact weight of that bag of clothing. It's not a good idea to try to weigh the bag of clothing alone on the scale. Most scales of this type don't do very well with such minimal weights on their platforms. Instead, get on the scale while holding the bag of clothes. (It doesn't matter what you're currently wearing during this operation.) Write down what you weigh while holding the bag of clothes. Then put the bag of clothes aside and weigh yourself again without it.

Are you getting the idea? The difference between the two weights is the weight of your weighing clothes in the bag. The only thing you want to remember about this outing is how much the weighing clothes alone weigh. Forget what you weigh at this time. You aren't currently wearing those weighing clothes.

Here's the important part. In the future, every time you weigh yourself on that very same scale, be sure you're wearing your weighing clothes. Weigh yourself then subtract what you know to be the weight of your weighing clothes. That's your nude weight, and you're not even nude.

The downside to this technique is that, in time, a store clerk may comment, "There goes the lady with the red blouse, the green skirt, and the purple shoes again. Does she only have one outfit?" I would assert that this is a minor price to pay for acquiring such valuable information.

*Chapter 20*

# Hunger Wrecks Diets

A nd now, the moment you've been waiting for. The "diet" part of this diet book. In this chapter and the next two, I'm going to give you information and explicit instructions that I guarantee will lead you to your goal weight provided that you (1) follow my advice under your doctor's supervision and (2) follow it to the letter (subject to any changes made to them by your doctor).

Before I get to the detailed, step-by-step instructions, I'm going to jump right to the punch line. I've condensed all that I've learned about losing weight during my 50-year medical career into one brief statement. Are you ready to be enlightened? Are you ready to learn the secret to losing weight? Here it is:

Eat less.

*"That's it?"* you ask incredulously. *"That's your brilliant advice?"*

Yes. The way to lose weight (that is, fat) is to take in fewer calories than you require to maintain your weight. Do you need me to be more specific? OK, I'll modify my instructions: eat 1,000 calories a day. So what's the problem? If it's that simple, why are approximately 65 percent of us overweight? Because on that treacherous road that runs between our best intentions and the treasure that is our ideal weight lurks a formidable highway bandit: hunger.

Everyone knows that the way to lose weight is to eat less. So pick a diet, any diet. I promise you it will work as long as it results in a caloric deficit. Oh, and you have to stick to it. Ah, there's the rub. The main reason that diets fail is that we're too hungry to follow them long enough to achieve the desired results.

If you're a "yo-yo dieter" who has tried and failed on this or that diet, you shouldn't feel guilty. It probably wasn't your fault. If the number of calories you were instructed to consume was low enough to produce meaningful weight loss in a reasonable period of time, then I can say with certainty that the hunger you experienced was extreme and, ultimately, unbearable. Hunger is a powerful sensation devised by Nature to keep the species going even during periods of great privation. Hunger has led men to war. Hunger has led men to kill. Hunger has even led men to eat processed, pasteurized cheese food product.

And so we've come to the crux of the matter, the Dr. Siegal's Cookie Diet *raison d'être*. The reason I've been so successful at helping people lose weight is that, back in 1975, I figured out how to control their hunger and enable them to stick to a low-calorie diet until they reached their goals. I feel that I owe you an explanation as to how I did it. After all, as you must have figured out by now, I'm about to ask you to make a leap of faith and trust me when I claim that you will lose weight—safely—by eating only cookies during the day and a modest dinner at night.

In the early 1970s, I was doing research for a book that I was writing on natural food substances that are particularly hunger suppressing. I knew from personal experience that some foods do a better job than others of controlling hunger and that some other foods actually stimulate hunger. Initially my research had a more theoretical than practical purpose, but that changed one day when I began to consider the possibility of trying to engineer a food specifically to control hunger. As far as I knew, nobody had ever done that before, and I don't know of anyone who has done so since.

My motivation to create a hunger-controlling food was my patients. I had been limiting my practice to the treatment of weight-related problems for 15 years, and while my success rate in getting the weight off my patients was higher than those of most of my fellow doctors, it still wasn't very high. Those who followed my advice lost weight but not enough followed my advice. They were simply too hungry.

I was fortunate to have had a strong chemistry background as well as a passion for cooking. I doubt I would have succeeded otherwise. I knew that the substance I hoped to create would be composed mainly of protein. It was already known at the time that protein was more satisfying of hunger than carbohydrates. Is there any doubt that a slab of BBQ ribs is more hunger controlling than a bowl of rice? The challenge I faced was that the most hunger-controlling foods were those that were high in fat (and, therefore, calories).

For several years, I experimented with various techniques for combining a blend of proteins that would result in a certain mixture of amino acids. Eventually I came up with a mixture of proteins that I was ready to put to the test. In order make it palatable, however, I needed to put my concoction into a food that someone would actually want to eat. As the world now knows, the first food I chose was a cookie. I wanted a food that didn't have to be prepared or refrigerated and that my patients, most of whom are female, could carry in their purses.

I baked the initial batches of cookies at home. My test subjects were my wife, my kids, and my neighbors. I instructed them to eat a cookie and tell me how it made them feel. Their answers were consistent. They said that the cookie left them less hungry than they would have expected from something so small. After a few more months of tinkering with the formula and with various flavors, I had the food I had set out to create. It was a 90 calorie oatmeal raisin cookie.

Sometime in 1975 I selected a small group of patients and offered them the opportunity to try a new diet. I told them that the diet would require them to eat just 1,200 calories per day and that they were to consume those calories exactly as I instructed. They were to eat six cookies per day, not at regular times but as needed to control hunger. Other than diet beverages and water, absolutely nothing else, not even a stick of gum, was to be consumed during the day. In the evening, they were to have a reasonable dinner consisting of six ounces of skinless chicken or turkey breast or non-fatty fish, prepared without oils, and one cup of non-starchy green vegetables.

Two weeks after I gave them their cookies and sent them on their way, my subjects began to return for their follow-up exams. After examining and talking with perhaps a dozen or so patients, I knew that my cookie offered enough hunger suppression to enable most people to adhere to a 1,200 calorie diet. I soon learned that I could go lower than 1,200 calories—a lot lower—and still keep hunger at bay. Eventually I concluded that 800 calories produces the fastest possible fat loss. But was it safe? Time would tell, and tell it did. Those early patients had no significant problems on my newfangled diet, and neither have any of the 500,000 who have followed them during the past 34 years.

To say that Dr. Siegal's Cookie Diet was an immediate success is an understatement. By the mid-1980s, my Miami medical practice had grown to include 14 clinics in Florida and 10 in Latin America. More than 200 other doctors throughout the United States were using my cookies in their own practices. The media and my patients had dubbed me "The Cookie Doctor."

So much for the history lesson. I want to get back to the instructions for the diet—*your* diet. First, however, I have to answer a question that I know you're dying to ask me: If I believe that 800 calories is the ideal daily caloric intake for achieving fat loss, why am I suggesting to your doctor and you that you follow a 1,000 calorie diet? The answer is that I'm not your doctor, I don't know your doctor, and I don't know your medical history. I know my own level of experience and expertise and that I'm qualified to determine which of my patients should be on an 800 calorie diet. If you want to follow an 800 calorie diet and want me to supervise you, feel free to call my office and schedule an appointment. (Be prepared to make monthly trips to South Florida.) If your doctor determines that you should be on an 800 calorie diet and is willing to supervise it, then that's your decision and his. My suggestion to both of you is that you follow a 1,000 calorie diet under his supervision.

There isn't a human being on the planet who can maintain her weight on 1,000 calories a day.[1] In fact, at that level, three out of four people lose about 10 pounds of fat per month. The rest lose weight too but, due to an easily corrected metabolic problem, they do it at a slower rate. If you suspect you are one of them, be sure to read Chapter 14.

I didn't pull that figure out of a hat. I based it on many years of experience with actual patients. I've had patients on diets ranging from 1,400 calories down to as few as 600. You might be surprised to know that people burn fat faster on 1,000 calories than on 600. I've learned that when you go much below 800 calories, the body goes into self-preservation mode. Your metabolism slows, and you begin to lose muscle and water in addition to fat. But within a range of 800 to 1,200 calories, your body burns fat at maximum efficiency and sheds pounds so fast that your motivation to continue is assured.

---

[1] That goes for 1,200 calories too, so don't be concerned if your doctor chooses to increase the suggested daily caloric intake a bit. Your weight-loss rate will be a little slower but it is still guaranteed.

Now that you know the secret to losing weight (eat less) and the primary reason diets fail (hunger), you're ready to begin losing weight with Dr. Siegal's Cookie Diet.

*Chapter 21*

# Dr. Siegal's Cookie Diet

## Three Steps to a Thinner, Healthier You

O K. You've read the preceding chapters and learned the long history and basic premise behind Dr. Siegal's Cookie Diet. You've obtained your doctor's permission to begin the diet and his consent to monitor you. So what are we waiting for? Let's get you to a healthful weight!

The weight-loss phase of your diet (I talk about weight maintenance in Chapter 22) consists of three steps that you must complete *in order:*

Step 1: Test your personal calorie burn rate as you lose weight for 28 days.

Step 2: Set your goal weight, and estimate when you'll reach it.

Step 3: Follow a reduced-calorie diet until you reach your goal weight.

## Dr. Siegal's Weight-Loss Calculators

Shortly before finishing this book, I decided to take the guesswork out of setting and reaching one's weight-loss goal. I designed several weight-loss calculators based on algorithms I had developed over the past few years. (Those college math classes finally paid off!) My mathematical formulas calculate with reasonable accuracy (this stuff isn't an exact science) the following data:

1.  The number of calories an individual's own body requires to maintain its weight.
2.  The number of days it will take to reach a goal weight eating a fixed number of calories each day.
3.  As an alternative to No. 2 above, the number of calories one would have to eat each day to reach a specified weight by a specified date (for example, to reach a weight of 125 pounds by June 1).

The three steps to losing weight on Dr. Siegal's Cookie Diet incorporate these calculators.

## Step 1: Check Your Metabolism as You Lose Weight

Everyone's metabolism is unique. We burn fat at different rates. On 1,800 calories, for example, you may lose five pounds per month while I gain three. It's absurd to think that everyone following a diet with a fixed number of calories will lose at the same rate. I'll bet you've tried diets that made that claim.

We're not going to repeat that mistake now. Instead, we're going to determine the approximate rate at which *your* body burns fat, and that will help you set a realistic, attainable goal.

Dr. Siegal's 28-day Calorie Burn Rate Self-test takes 28 days to complete. Unlike most tests, however, you don't have to complete this one before you start to lose weight. On the contrary, you'll start burning fat on the very first day.

During the 28 day test period, you'll eat a fixed number of calories every day. I suggest 1,000 calories, but your doctor may dictate more or less. Always take his advice. As long as the total number of calories is no more than 1,400, the test will yield useful results, and you'll lose weight. To deal with hunger, you'll eat Dr. Siegal's Cookie Diet cookies, shakes, or both. In the evening you'll have a satisfying dinner. You'll weigh yourself on the first and last days of the test. Then you'll enter your starting and ending weights, your activity level, and your fixed daily caloric intake, into a free calculator located in the Resources section of CookieDiet.com. (If you don't have Internet access, call 877-377-4342 (from North America) or 001 703-677-8068 (from elsewhere) to do the calculation by phone at no charge.)

The calculator, called Dr. Siegal's Calorie Burn Rate Calculator, will estimate how many calories your body requires each day to maintain your weight. Armed with that number, you'll then use one of two Dr. Siegal's Weight-Loss Goal Calculators to estimate the date on which you can expect to reach your desired weight based on a predetermined daily caloric intake. Alternatively, this flexible tool will tell you how many calories you would have to consume each day (with your doctor's approval) in order to reach your desired weight by a specific date (such as a wedding, high school reunion, or summer vacation).

*In order to take Dr. Siegal's 28-day Calorie Burn Rate Self-test, you'll need a one-month supply (four Weekly Boxes) of Dr. Siegal's Cookie Diet cookies, shake mixes, or a combination of the two. You can buy them on CookieDiet.com, by phone, or at a local retailer. To order by phone or to find a retailer near you, call CookieDiet.com. Contact information is provided under Notices at the beginning of the book.*

## Dr. Siegal's Calorie Burn Rate Self-test

As soon as you awaken in the morning on the first day of the test, weigh yourself in the nude, after going to the bathroom.

Write down your weight and store the number where you'll be able find it 28 days from then. For the next 28 days, eat six Dr. Siegal's Cookie Diet cookies (one shake may be substituted for two cookies) throughout the day but absolutely no other food except water and diet beverages. In the evening have a reasonable dinner as described later in this chapter.

After weighing yourself on the morning of the 28th day, determine your daily calorie burn rate using the free Dr. Siegal's Calorie Burn Rate Calculator. To do this online, go to CookieDiet.com. If you're already a registered user, log in and go to the Resources section. Otherwise, create a new free account. After logging in, follow the simple instructions to calculate your results.

If you don't have Internet access, you can obtain your Daily Caloric Maintenance Level for free by phone. Call the CookieDiet.com toll-free number and choose the option for Consumer Relations. A support specialist will enter your information into the calculator and give you the results.

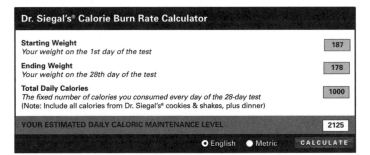

*Dr. Siegal's Calorie Burn Rate Calculator estimates your Daily Caloric Maintenance Level*

## Step 2: Set Your Goal

After completing Step 1, you're ready to set your weight-loss goal. In almost every field of human endeavor, it's easier to reach a goal that is clearly defined. Weight loss is no exception. That's why I'm going to give you an easy way to set a realistic, attainable weight-loss goal in addition to showing you how to reach it.

You may have set goals on previous diets, but my guess is that you simply picked a number of pounds you hoped to lose, say 40 pounds, and hoped for the best. Perhaps you got a little more specific by adding a time frame (to lose the 40 pounds by summer or something like that). Unfortunately, in previous attempts to lose weight, you probably gave little thought to whether your goal was realistic. I'm sure your enthusiasm was there. But by realistic, I mean mathematically possible. It's axiomatic that you'll burn fat if you eat less than you need to maintain your weight. But there's a limit to how fast you can lose fat, even on a very-low-calorie diet. What's the limit, you ask? It's about 10 pounds per month. Anyone who sheds pounds much faster than that probably loses muscle and water as well.

As I mentioned earlier, I have developed weight-loss calculators to help you set a realistic goal. These calculators offer two methods of goal setting:

**Method 1: Fixed Calories.** You specify the fixed number of calories you wish to eat each day, and the calculator will estimate the date on which you will reach your goal weight at that calorie level. This method is best if you're more concerned with the quantity of food you'll eat each day than the length of time it will take to reach your goal.

**Method 2: Weight by Date.** You specify the date on which you want to reach your goal weight, and the calculator will estimate how many calories you'd need to consume each day to reach your goal by that date. This method is best if your goal is to "look your best" for a special occasion and you're flexible as to the fixed amount of food you'll eat each day. With this method, if the date of your event is far in the future or the amount of weight you need to lose is small, the amount of calories may be much higher than 1,000. For example, if you want to lose only 20 pounds in six months, you'll probably

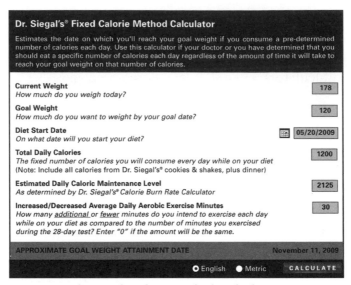

*Dr. Siegal's Fixed Calorie Method Calculator estimates the date on which you will reach your goal weight if you consume a specified number of calories each day*

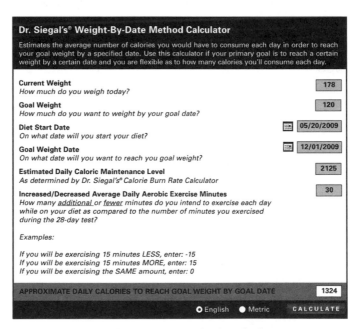

*Dr. Siegal's Weight-By-Date Method Calculator estimates how many calories you would have to consume each day to reach your goal weight by a specific date*

be able to achieve that goal by eating 1,400 to 1,800 calories a day. The calculators have built-in safeguards that prevent them from displaying unrealistic or unhealthful values. If your goal is unattainable, the calculators will say so. You won't be given false hope.

## Step 3: Reach Your Goal Weight

This step is actually a continuation of Step 1. Continue to use Dr. Siegal's Cookie Diet cookies and shakes during the day to satisfy hunger. Have a compatible dinner in the evening as described next.

As you now know, the plan is for you to eat Dr. Siegal's cookies during the day at times when hunger strikes and eat a dinner later in the day. The dinner adds to the 500 calories that came from the six cookies.

That dinner may originate from various sources, not unlike the dinners you currently eat. You may prepare it from scratch, you may eat it in a restaurant, or you may buy it ready-made and bring it home or have it delivered. Which of these is most likely to have a positive result, one that will supply you with the right amount and kinds of nutrients?

On the surface it would seem that home cooking is the answer. That way you can choose the exact items and the exact amounts that will go into your dinner. In practice, it's not that clear. Have you ever prepared dinner for one person? Combining a slew of ingredients in very small quantities generally feels as though it isn't worth the trouble. It's easier to order in a pizza. The latter is definitely not the way to go.

Restaurant food could be the answer if the staff could provide precisely what you want. What are the chances that would happen?

Let's not belabor the point. Frozen dinners from the supermarket meet the need. There are a variety of them, and some actually come very close to my requirements. What's that? You say that's not your favorite way to have dinner? Wasn't it your preferred way that contributed to your problem?

*Read this section only if you plan to follow a 1,000 calorie diet.*

# Frozen Dinners: 1,000 Calorie Diet

There is no question that frozen dinners are a convenient way to facilitate your diet. Anything that makes your task a little easier is welcome. What we sacrifice with frozen dinners is perfection. We can't always get the exact mix of protein, carbohydrate, and fat that would be desirable, but we gain convenience. Anything that keeps you on the diet is OK with me.

Since I always strive for what is practical, I think that reasonable use of frozen dinners is likely to keep you on track. One real advantage to eating them is that you really know what nutrients you're getting; they're printed on the package. I'm sure you're familiar with the "diet" type of frozen dinners, brands such as Lean Cuisine and Healthy Choice. They are actually too low in calories for our 1,000 calorie diet. Most of them are about 350 calories or less. Add that to the 500 calories that you will get from my cookies and you have only an 850 calorie diet. Don't fret. I have what is probably going to be very good news.

In order to get enough calories to meet the requirement of a 500 calorie dinner, you are going to need two frozen dinners of this type. Yes, you heard me right—two frozen dinners. This could really be a historical first—two dinners required for a super-fast reducing diet. The idea is to have 500 calories for dinner, so two dinners of about 250 calories each will do it quite nicely.

Stop jumping for joy and hear me out. There are several brands of frozen diet dinners out there, and the only real reason to choose one brand over another has to do with the Nutrition Facts panel on the box. If the numbers add up correctly, that's all that counts. Therefore, you could have two identical dinners, or if you prefer variety, two different dinners.

There are two numbers on that Nutrition Facts panel that you need to become friends with: calories per serving and protein content. Every package has these values printed prominently. The calories per serving we are striving for is 500. Your two choices have to add up to 500, give or take 20 or 30 calories. Just as important is the amount of protein. Remember, protein helps with hunger. The total protein in your two dinners together should be at least 30 grams. If those two requirements are met, go for it.

It would be nice if I could list every eligible frozen diet dinner, but it's impossible. The manufacturers change the lineup so frequently that it would lead to frustration. Furthermore, they sometimes change the recipe for a particular item without warning; the only way to know is to read the Nutrition Facts panel. Don't ever assume that the package you've just picked out of the freezer case has the same nutrients as it did the last time you bought it.

I'm going to list only a few to serve as examples. I've chosen them from the very popular brands, those that are in virtually every supermarket. It's not that I prefer these particularly; they are simply examples. Don't forget to *read the Nutrition Facts panel.*

| | Calories Per Serving | Protein (grams) |
|---|---|---|
| Stouffer's Lean Cuisine Shrimp Alfredo | 260 | 18 |
| Healthy Choice Grilled Chicken Marinara | 250 | 20 |
| Healthy Choice Grilled Whiskey Steak | 250 | 18 |
| Stouffer's Lean Cuisine Meatloaf & Whipped Potatoes | 260 | 21 |
| Stouffer's Lean Cuisine Alfredo Pasta with Chicken & Broccoli | 250 | 17 |
| Healthy Choice Cajun Style Chicken & Shrimp | 250 | 18 |
| Stouffer's Lean Cuisine Chicken Pecan | 260 | 19 |
| Healthy Choice Creamy Dill Salmon | 240 | 19 |
| Stouffer's Lean Cuisine Chicken Mediterranean | 240 | 19 |

There are not many single frozen dinners (not the diet brands) in the 500 calorie range. Here are a few, but most miss the mark in calories or protein. Still, you may have them as long as you don't make a habit of them. Remember to eat only one of these, not two.

|  | Calories Per Serving | Protein (grams) |
|---|---|---|
| Marie Callender's Meatloaf & Gravy | 560 | 31 |
| Marie Callender's Herb Roasted Chicken and Mashed Potato | 530 | 34 |
| Stouffer's Chicken Monterey | 500 | 28 |
| Stouffer's Salisbury Steak | 470 | 29 |

*Skip to page 230, "Home Cooking."*

**Read this section only if you plan to follow a 1,200 calorie diet.**

# Frozen Dinners: 1,200 Calorie Diet

There is no question that frozen dinners are a convenient way to facilitate your diet. Anything that makes your task a little easier is welcome. What we sacrifice with frozen dinners is perfection. We can't always get the exact mix of protein, carbohydrate, and fat that would be desirable, but we gain convenience. Anything that keeps you on the diet is OK with me.

Since I always strive for what is practical, I think that reasonable use of frozen dinners is likely to keep you on track. One real advantage to eating them is that you really know what nutrients you're getting; they're printed on the package. I'm sure you are familiar with the "diet" type of frozen dinners, brands such as Lean Cuisine and Healthy Choice. They are actually too low in calories for our 1,200 calorie diet. Most of them are about 350 calories or less. Add that to the 500 calories that you will get from my cookies and you have only an 850 calorie diet. Don't fret. I have what is probably going to be very good news.

In order to get enough calories to meet the requirement of a 700 calorie dinner, you are going to need two frozen dinners. Yes, you heard me right—two frozen dinners. This could really be a historical first—two dinners required for a super-fast reducing diet. The idea is to have 700 calories for dinner, so two dinners of about 350 calories each will do it quite nicely.

Stop jumping for joy and hear me out. There are several brands of frozen diet dinners out there, and the only real reason to prefer one brand over another has to do with the Nutrition Facts panel on the box. If the numbers add up correctly, that's all that counts. Therefore, you could have two identical dinners, or if you prefer variety, two different dinners.

There are two numbers on that Nutrition Facts panel that you need to become friends with: calories per serving and protein content. Every package has these values printed prominently. The calories per serving we are striving for is 700. Your two choices have to add up to 700, give or take 20 or 30 calories. Just as important is the amount of protein. Remember, protein helps with hunger. The total protein of your two dinners together should be at least 45 grams. If those two requirements are met, go for it.

It would be nice if I could list every possible frozen diet dinner here, but it's impossible. The manufacturers change the lineup so frequently that it would lead to frustration. Furthermore, they sometimes change the recipe for a particular item without warning; the only way to know is to read the Nutrition Facts panel. Don't ever assume that the package you've just picked out of the freezer case has the same nutrients as it did the last time you bought it.

I'm going to list only a few to serve as examples. I've chosen them from very popular brands, those that are in virtually every supermarket. It's not that I prefer these particularly; they are simply examples. Don't forget to *read the Nutrition Facts panel.*

| | Calories Per Serving | Protein (grams) |
|---|---|---|
| Stouffer's LeanCuisine Pesto Chicken with Bow Tie Pasta | 340 | 23 |
| Weight Watchers Smart Ones Bistro Selections Chicken Fettuccini | 340 | 23 |
| Healthy Choice Chicken Margherita | 340 | 23 |
| Stouffer's Lean Cuisine Chicken Club Panini | 350 | 24 |
| Stouffer's Lean Cuisine Balsamic Glazed Chicken | 350 | 24 |

## Home Cooking

Who would dare disparage home cooking? I would. Cooking your diet dinner at home of course gives you the most versatility, the most chance to get it exactly right, doesn't it? You can put the exact amount you wish into the pot and you know that if the goal is to have a 500 calorie dinner, you can actually control it. Not so fast. Yes, you can do it if you have the right data, but where is that going to come from? The U.S. Department of Agriculture has done an amazing job of evaluating every possible food for nutrient content, calories, carbohydrate, protein, and much more. If your interest is meat, and specifically a particular cut such as beef round, you can find all the information on their Web site. It shouldn't be too hard to decipher. Well, guess how many entries are under "beef round." There are 123. Can you believe that? To show you the complexity of all this, here are just eight of the 123. Read them then forget them.

– *Beef, round, bottom round, separable lean only, trimmed to 1/8" fat, choice, raw*

– *Beef, round, full cut separable lean and fat, trimmed to 1/8" fat, select, raw*

- *Beef , round, outside round, bottom round, steak, separable lean and fat, trimmed to 0" fat, all grades, raw*

- *Beef, round, outside round, bottom round, steak, separable lean and fat, trimmed to 0" fat, choice, raw*

- *Beef, round, tip round, separable lean and fat trimmed to 0" fat, all grades, raw*

- *Beef, round, tip round, separable lean and fat, trimmed to 1/8" fat, all grades, raw*

- *Beef, round, top round, separable lean only, trimmed to 1/8" fat, all grades, raw*

- *Beef, round, top round, separable lean only, trimmed to 1/8" fat, select, raw*

This goes on and on. Each has its own values for calories, carbohydrate, fat, and a host of other nutrients. And the values differ broadly, even though they are all "beef, round." When you select your meat at the supermarket, when you pick up that package of beef round steak, how can you possibly know which of the 123 entries under "beef, round" you are holding in your hand? And even if you could make an intelligent guess, can you be sure that the cow that contributed to that package had the same dietary history as the one that they tested in the laboratory? It's impossible. You'd be lucky to guess the nutrition of that hunk of meat within 50 percent of the actual values. Of course, you could spend a bundle sending it to a laboratory for analysis, but then your dinner would be gone.

When you get to the supermarket, are you really going to know the grade of beef, whether there is 1/8" of fat, etc.? Do you know that after you cook it, all the nutritional information changes? Again, forget it.

So why did I go to the trouble of giving you such detailed information if it is not at all helpful? I don't want you to waste your time doing a fruitless task. I know you're serious about making this program work, so I'm going to tell you how to do it.

If you're determined to cook your own meat dinner, select meat that looks as lean as possible, and if it has visible fat, trim it off and discard it. Cook the meat well by either frying (without fat) or stewing or roasting. Accompany it with the quantity of vegetables specified below. Flavor it with dry spices to your liking. If your doctor has warned you about salt, heed his advice. Use the following amounts based on the number of calories you want to take in per day:

### 1,000 calorie diet:

A 500 calorie dinner containing six ounces of cooked beef
Vegetables should make up 100 more calories (see lists below)

### 1,200 calorie diet:

A 700 calorie dinner containing 7.5 ounces of cooked beef
Vegetables should make up 200 more calories (see lists below)

Will that give you exactly what I want you to have? No, not exactly but it's good enough. Remember, I take the practical approach. Some people just love to cook. I'm assuming that you're not going to do this every day. A few times a month will not make a big difference.

If you want to use chicken in place of beef, make sure it's boneless breast without skin. Substitute it for beef in the above.

### 1,000 calorie diet:

A 500 calorie dinner containing eight ounces of cooked chicken breast
Vegetables should make up 100 more calories (see list below)

### 1,200 calorie diet:

A 700 calorie dinner containing 10 ounces of cooked chicken breast
Vegetables should make up 200 more calories (see list below)

# Other Sources of Protein

The deli counter at the supermarket and the packaged cold cuts section are sources of allowed protein. Products such as packaged turkey breast or even ham can be used. Fortunately, the packages list the calories and protein content. Remember your requirements as listed above and eat just that amount. The nutritional labels of the packaged products can serve as a guideline for the virtually identical products at the deli counter. If you ask, they'll slice exact quantities (one-meal portions) for your convenience.

## Tuna

Tuna is a good source of protein. Of course, fresh tuna is great, but it's also available in cans and sealed pouches. Make sure it's packed in water, not oil. There are 5- and 12-ounce cans. A whole 5-ounce can has 150 calories and about 30 grams of protein.

## Other Fish and Seafood

I do know that tuna is a fish, but I have listed it separately because it is so readily available. It's in a special class.

There are many choices in fish and seafood, and I wouldn't mind a bit if you concentrated on them. I'd prefer the following very-low-fat seafood:

| | | |
|---|---|---|
| clams | oysters | sole |
| crab, all varieties | perch | whiting |
| flounder | orange roughy | |
| grouper | pike | |
| haddock | pollock | |
| halibut | sea bass | |
| lobster | snapper | |

Note: The protein content of this group is 5 to 6 grams per ounce. (Clams are a little less.) Catfish, mussels, and smelt have a little more fat, but you may have them on occasion. On rare occasions you may have the really fatty fish such as salmon, mackerel, lake trout, or herring.

## Egg White (one of my favorites)

You can always be shamefully wasteful by cracking open eggs and discarding the yolks. But there is another way, and you won't feel guilty. Egg whites come already separated from the yolks and are sold in refrigerated cartons. In the supermarket are also one or more brands of "egg substitutes" (e.g., Egg Beaters) that are really egg whites flavored to taste like whole eggs. Both of these products are acceptable. The different brands of each vary slightly in calories and protein. It will be a test of your culinary skills to utilize them to your advantage by combining them with other foods.

For about 100 calories from packaged egg whites, you'll need about 3/4 cup of them, which will give you about 20 grams of protein.

You may want to try this 250 calorie omelet with lots of protein. Alone, it is not enough for dinner. You'll have to supplement it with other foods such as frozen dinners.

First sauté (dry) in a skillet a nice selection of veggies such as mushrooms, onions, peppers, and spices. (See the list below.) Then add a cup of egg whites. If you like, mix in a couple of tablespoons of cottage cheese. (There's not that much difference between the regular stuff and the 2 percent milkfat variety.) You'll be on your way to a big omelet. If you prefer, you can use one of the egg substitutes to get about the same result. Warning: since you're not adding any oil, use a nonstick skillet.

# Shrimp

This is another of my favorites because of the high-quality protein and its availability. Many supermarkets have refrigerated (or frozen) cleaned, cooked shrimp available in two or more sizes. It is quite convenient to cook them into various dishes or to eat them cold with not much more than a trace of cocktail sauce or lemon juice. You'll be amazed at how many shrimp are allowed. The only negative is that your doctor may have his own ideas on the subject of shrimp and cholesterol. Ask.

For 100 calories and 18 grams of protein, you will need about 3 ounces of shrimp. That's equivalent to about 8 medium-sized or 5 extra-large shrimp. You can see that a 400 calorie portion of them would involve an impressive amount of shrimp, possibly more than you'd care to have at a meal. Consider a 100 calorie or 200 calorie portion as an appetizer to be supplemented with an appropriate frozen dinner or home-cooked dish.

# Vegetables

I'm sure you can guess which are allowed. Concentrate on the green ones and forget the starchy ones. Potatoes, corn, and rice are out.[1]

Here are two vegetable lists. The first is labeled "any reasonable amount." What more can I say about that? I guess it's possible to overdose on lettuce, but who would want to? The second list specifies quantities. Remember the nutritional content of foods is quite variable. Use this list as a guideline. If you want something that is not listed, consult the Internet or one of those calorie books.

---

[1] Don't remind me that I'm inconsistent. I already know it, but I have an explanation. Since the nutrient content of these forbidden substances is taken into account by the manufacturers of packaged and frozen foods, I'll allow you to have them. But let's leave those calculations to the professionals.

Neither is great but they're better than just a wild guess. Don't agonize over what constitutes "medium" or "large."

Of course, it's permissible to mix vegetables, but the choices will depend on whether you need a 100 calorie or 200 calorie portion.

Since all the quantities listed are for raw vegetables, it is very important that you add no fat or oil in the cooking process.

As for canned or frozen vegetables, they are allowed. Consult the label for quantities and calorie counts.

### Vegetables, raw, any reasonable amount

Asparagus
Green beans
Celery
Cucumber
Green peppers
Lettuce
Mushrooms
Radishes
Rhubarb
Spinach

### Vegetables, raw, 100 calorie portions

| | |
|---|---|
| Broccoli | 2 small stalks |
| Cabbage | 1/2 head |
| Carrots | 2 medium |
| Cauliflower | 1/2 large head |
| Eggplant | about 1 peeled |
| Green peas | 1 cup |
| Onions | 2 cups sliced |
| Parsnips | 1 cup |
| Tomatoes, ripe | 3 large |
| Turnips | 2 large |
| Zucchini | 2 large |

# Recipes

If you really enjoy being a chef, here's your chance. These 500 calorie and 700 calorie recipes that each provide four servings. You may use them for a family meal (or increase the quantity if you have a bigger family).

You may also choose to prepare these recipes and freeze them to create your own frozen dinners. Divide each into four portions and freeze them in plastic bags or reusable containers.

These recipes are not chiseled in stone. They are here to serve as a guide or an example of what you may have for dinner. You can vary them within reason. Of course, you don't want to seriously alter the calorie count. For example, don't drop a quarter pound of butter into the pot.

## 500 Calorie Dinner Menu
### *Basil Shrimp*

*4 servings*

1 lb raw shrimp, peeled and deveined

1/4 tsp salt

¼ tsp cayenne pepper

1/4 tsp ground turmeric

1 Tbsp extra virgin olive oil

1 bunch scallions, rough chopped

1/4 c firmly packed basil leaves, finely chopped

1 tsp fresh-squeezed lemon juice

*Preparation:*

1. Season shrimp with salt, cayenne pepper, and turmeric in a medium bowl. Cover and let marinate for 30 minutes in the refrigerator.

2. Heat olive oil in large nonstick skillet over medium-high heat. Cook shrimp about one minute on high then turn them over and cook an additional minute.
3. To skillet, add scallions and basil and cook for 1 to 2 minutes, stirring constantly. Shrimp are thoroughly cooked when they turn pink.
4. Add lemon juice and serve.

*\* Add mango or pineapple for a Caribbean flavor, if desired*

### Cherry Tomato Bean Salad
### Dressed in Basil Vinaigrette

*4 servings*

1/4 lb green beans, trimmed

1/4 lb yellow beans, trimmed

1/8 c good-quality balsamic vinegar

1 tsp extra virgin olive oil

1/4 tsp kosher salt

1/4 tsp freshly ground pepper

1-1/2 c cherry tomatoes, halved

1/4 c firmly packed basil leaves, chopped

1/4 c red onion, chopped

*Preparation:*
1. Add beans to a pot of boiling water and cook for 5 minutes. Drain beans and submerge in ice water for 1 minute then drain.
2. In a bowl, combine balsamic vinegar, oil, salt, and pepper. Wisk mixture together.
3. Add beans, tomatoes, basil leaves, and onion to mixture.
4. Toss dressing in bowl and let chill in the refrigerator for an hour.

# 700 Calorie Dinner Menu
## *Basil Shrimp*

*4 servings*

1-1/2 lb raw shrimp, peeled and deveined

1/2 tsp salt

1/2 tsp cayenne pepper

1/2 tsp ground turmeric

1 Tbsp extra virgin olive oil

1 bunch scallions, rough chopped

1 ripe mango, peeled and cut into 1/2-inch cubes*

1/4 c firmly packed basil leaves, finely chopped

1 tsp fresh-squeezed lemon juice

*Preparation:*

1. Season shrimp with salt, cayenne pepper, and turmeric in a medium bowl. Cover and let marinate for 30 minutes in the refrigerator.
2. Heat olive oil in large nonstick skillet over medium-high heat. Cook shrimp about one minute on and turn them over and cook an additional minute.
3. To skillet, add scallions and basil and cook for 1 to 2 minutes, stirring constantly. Shrimp are thoroughly cooked when they turn pink.
4. Add lemon juice and serve.

\* *You can use pineapple instead, if desired*

## *Cherry Tomato Bean Salad*

*4 servings*

1/2 lb green beans, trimmed

1/2 lb yellow beans, trimmed

1/8 c good-quality balsamic vinegar

1 tsp extra virgin olive oil

1/4 tsp Kosher salt

1/4 tsp freshly ground pepper

1-1/2 c cherry tomatoes, halved

1/2 c of firmly packed basil leaves, chopped

1/4 c red onion, chopped

*Preparation:*
1. Add beans to a pot of boiling water and cook for 5 minutes. Drain beans and rinse in cold water.
2. In a bowl, combine balsamic vinegar, oil, salt, and pepper. Wisk mixture together.
3. Add beans, tomatoes, basil leaves, and onion to mixture.
4. Toss dressing in bowl and let chill in the refrigerator for an hour. Serve.

# 500 Calorie Dinner Menu
## *Chicken Breast Topped with Goat Cheese Bruschetta*

*4 servings*

2 c chopped tomato

1/3 c chopped onion

1/3 c fresh basil, chopped

2 tsp extra virgin olive oil

2 tsp balsamic vinegar

1 tsp Kosher salt

4 (6 oz) chicken breasts, boneless and skinless

1/4 tsp freshly ground black pepper

Cooking spray

3 Tbsp reduced-fat goat cheese, crumbled

*Preparation:*

1. Combine tomato, onion, basil, olive oil, vinegar, and half the salt in a medium bowl.
2. Gently pound chicken breasts to 1-inch thickness using a meat mallet.
3. Sprinkle both sides of chicken with remaining salt and pepper.
4. Heat a large nonstick skillet over medium-high heat. Coat pan with cooking spray. Cook chicken breasts until chicken is browned and done. Use a meat thermometer to ensure doneness; chicken should be 165°F.
5. Add feta cheese into tomato mixture and top chicken with about 1/2 cup of the goat cheese bruschetta mixture.

\* *You can substitute reduced-fat feta or gorgonzola cheese for the reduced-fat goat cheese, if desired*

### *Rosemary-infused Asparagus*

*4 servings*

1 lb asparagus

1 tsp olive oil

2 garlic cloves, minced

1 sprig rosemary

1/2 c water

1/2 tsp salt

1/4 tsp freshly ground black pepper

*Preparation:*

1. Rinse and dry asparagus. Prepare them by cutting off ends of the spears.
2. Heat olive oil in a large nonstick skillet over medium-high heat.
3. To the skillet, add asparagus, garlic, and rosemary and sauté 3 minutes or until asparagus is lightly browned.
4. Add 1/2 cup water to pan; cook 5 minutes or until asparagus is crisp-tender. The water in the pan should be almost gone.
5. Season asparagus with salt and pepper to taste and serve.

* *You can substitute broccoli for asparagus, if desired*

# 700 Calorie Dinner Menu
## *Chicken Breast Topped with Goat Cheese Bruschetta*

*4 servings*

2 c chopped tomato

1/3 c chopped onion

1/3 c fresh basil, chopped

2 tsp extra virgin olive oil

2 tsp balsamic vinegar

1 tsp kosher salt

4 (7 oz) chicken breasts, boneless and skinless

1/4 tsp freshly ground black pepper

Cooking spray

4 Tbsp reduced-fat goat cheese, crumbled

*Preparation:*

1. Combine tomato, onion, basil, olive oil, vinegar, and half the salt in a medium bowl.
2. Gently pound chicken breasts to 1-inch thickness using a meat mallet.
3. Sprinkle both sides of chicken with remaining salt and pepper.
4. Heat a large nonstick skillet over medium-high heat. Coat pan with cooking spray. Cook chicken breasts until chicken is browned and done. Use a meat thermometer to ensure doneness; chicken should be 165°F.
5. Add feta cheese into tomato mixture and top chicken with about 1/2 cup of the goat cheese bruschetta mixture.

\* *You can substitute reduced-fat feta or gorgonzola cheese for the reduced-fat goat cheese, if desired*

### *Rosemary-infused Asparagus*

*4 servings*

1 lb asparagus

1 tsp olive oil

2 garlic cloves, minced

1 sprig rosemary

1/2 c water

1/2 tsp salt

1/4 tsp freshly ground black pepper

*Preparation:*

1. Rinse and dry asparagus. Prepare them by cutting off ends of the spears.
2. Heat olive oil in a large nonstick skillet over medium-high heat.
3. To the skillet, add asparagus, garlic, and rosemary and sauté 3 minutes or until asparagus is lightly browned.
4. Add 1/2 cup water to pan; cook 5 minutes or until asparagus is crisp-tender. The water in the pan should be almost gone.
5. Season asparagus with salt and pepper to taste and serve.

*You can substitute broccoli for asparagus, if desired.

# 500 Calorie Dinner Menu
## *Tuna Steak with Soy Ginger Sauce*

*4 servings*

4 (6 oz) tuna fillets

4 Tbsp low-sodium soy sauce, divided

4 Tbsp rice wine vinegar

2 Tbsp freshly grated ginger

Cooking spray

Freshly ground pepper to taste

*Preparation:*

1. Marinate tuna with half each of the soy sauce, rice wine vinegar, and ginger. Leave in refrigerator for 30 minutes.
2. Wisk together remaining soy sauce, rice wine vinegar, and ginger. Set aside.
3. Heat grill pan over medium-high heat, and coat with cooking spray.
4. Season tuna steaks with pepper. Cook tuna for 2 minutes on each side, top with soy ginger sauce, and continue to cook to desired degree of doneness.

* *Add 2 tablespoons wasabi paste for additional Asian flavor, if desired*

** *Alternative cooking method: Heat 1 teaspoon of olive oil in 12-inch nonstick frying pan on high heat. Add tuna steaks and cook to desired degree of doneness.*

## *Asian-inspired Spinach*

*4 servings*

1-1/2 lb fresh spinach

1/2 tsp dark sesame oil

1 c scallions, chopped

3/4 tsp sesame seeds

1/2 tsp low-sodium soy sauce

2 tsp minced garlic

*Preparation:*
1. Wash and dry spinach thoroughly and trim the stems.
2. In large sauté pan, heat sesame oil over high heat until very hot.
3. Add spinach and cook for 1 to 2 minutes, stirring constantly.
4. Add to pan scallions, sesame seeds, soy sauce, and garlic; continue cooking spinach for an additional 30 seconds. Spinach should turn green and wilt.
5. Remove from heat, toss gently, and serve.

# 700 Calorie Dinner Menu
## *Tuna Steak with Soy Ginger Sauce*

*4 servings*

4 (7 oz) tuna fillets

4 Tbsp low-sodium soy sauce, divided

4 Tbsp rice wine vinegar

2 Tbsp freshly grated ginger

Cooking spray

Freshly ground pepper to taste

*Preparation:*

1. Marinate tuna with half each of the soy sauce, rice wine vinegar, and ginger. Leave in refrigerator for 30 minutes.
2. Wisk together remaining soy sauce, rice wine vinegar, and ginger. Set aside.
3. Heat grill pan on medium-high heat, and coat with cooking spray.
4. Season tuna steaks with pepper. Cook tuna for 2 minutes on each side, top with soy ginger sauce, and continue to cook to desired degree of doneness.

* Add 2 tablespoons wasabi paste for additional Asian flavor, if desired

**Alternative cooking method: Heat 1 teaspoon of olive oil in 12-inch nonstick frying pan on high heat. Add tuna steaks and cook to desired degree of doneness.*

### *Asian-inspired Spinach*

*4 servings*

2 lb fresh spinach

1/2 tsp dark sesame oil

1 c scallions, chopped

3/4 tsp sesame seeds

1/2 tsp low-sodium soy sauce

2 tsp minced garlic

Preparation:

1.  Wash and dry spinach thoroughly and trim stems.
2.  In large sauté pan, heat sesame oil over high heat until very hot.
3.  Add spinach and cook for 1 to 2 minutes, stirring constantly.
4.  To pan add scallions, sesame seeds, soy sauce, and garlic; continue cooking spinach for an additional 30 seconds. Spinach should turn green and wilt.
5.  Remove from heat, toss gently, and serve.

# 500 Calorie Dinner Menu
## *Tilapia in Lemon Dill Sauce*

*4 servings*

1/2 c fat-free, reduced-sodium chicken broth

1/4 c fresh-squeezed lemon juice

1 tsp grated lemon zest

3/4 Tbsp cornstarch

1 Tbsp minced parsley

1/4 tsp salt

1/8 tsp dried oregano

1/8 tsp dried rosemary

1/2 tsp freshly ground black pepper

Cooking spray

4 (6 oz) tilapia fillets

1 Tbsp minced fresh dill (or 1/2 tsp dried)

*Preparation:*

1. In a small saucepan, combine chicken broth, lemon juice, lemon zest, and cornstarch. Bring mixture to a boil, and cook for 1 minute, stirring constantly. Remove from heat. Stir in parsley, salt, oregano, rosemary, and pepper.
2. Heat a large nonstick skillet over medium-high heat. Coat skillet with cooking spray and cook fish one minute on each side. Add broth mixture and bring to a boil. Cover, reduce heat and simmer for an additional 5 to 7 minutes. Use a thermometer to ensure doneness; fish should be 145°F.
3. Remove fish from pan, and add dill to sauce. Stir for 1 minute. Serve approximately 2 tablespoons of sauce over fish.

### Brown Sugar Glazed Carrots

*4 servings*

1 tsp margarine

1/4 c packed brown sugar

1 tsp cornstarch

4 c sliced carrots

1/4 tsp salt

1/4 tsp freshly ground black pepper

1 pinch cinnamon

1 Tbsp water

1/4 c fresh parsley, chopped

*Preparation:*

1. In a large nonstick skillet, melt margarine and brown sugar over medium-high heat. Add cornstarch. It should turn into a glaze. Reduce heat to medium.
2. Add carrots, salt, and pepper to the skillet, and cook for an additional 10 minutes or until tender.
3. Sprinkle with cinnamon, top with parsley, and serve.

# 700 Calorie Dinner Menu
## *Tilapia in Lemon Dill Sauce*

### *4 servings*

1/2 c fat-free, reduced-sodium chicken broth

1/4 c fresh-squeezed lemon juice

1 tsp grated lemon zest

3/4 Tbsp cornstarch

1 Tbsp minced parsley

1/4 tsp salt

1/8 tsp dried oregano

1/8 tsp dried rosemary

1/2 tsp freshly ground black pepper

Cooking spray

4 (7 oz) tilapia fillets

1 Tbsp minced fresh dill (or 1/2 tsp dried)

*Preparation:*
1. In a small saucepan, combine chicken broth, lemon juice, lemon zest, and cornstarch. Bring mixture to a boil, and cook for 1 minute, stirring constantly. Remove from heat. Stir in parsley, salt, oregano, rosemary, and pepper.
2. Heat a large nonstick skillet over medium-high heat. Coat skillet with cooking spray, and cook fish one minute on each side. Add broth mixture and bring to a boil. Cover, reduce heat, and simmer for an additional 5 to 7 minutes. Use a thermometer to ensure doneness; fish should be 145°F.
3. Remove fish from pan and add dill to sauce. Stir for 1 minute. Serve approximately 2 tablespoons of sauce over fish.

### Brown Sugar Glazed Carrots

*4 servings*

1 tsp margarine

1/4 c packed brown sugar

1 tsp cornstarch

4-1/2 c sliced carrots

1/4 tsp salt

1/4 tsp freshly ground black pepper

1 Tbsp water

1 pinch cinnamon

1/4 c fresh parsley, chopped

*Preparation:*
1. In a large nonstick skillet, melt margarine and brown sugar over medium-high heat. Add cornstarch. It should turn into a glaze. Reduce heat to medium.
2. Add carrots, salt, and pepper to the skillet and cook for an additional 10 minutes or until tender.
3. Sprinkle with cinnamon, top with parsley, and serve.

# 500 Calorie Dinner Menu
## *Chicken Marsala*

*4 servings*

4 (6 oz) boneless, skinless chicken breasts

1/4 tsp salt

1/4 tsp freshly ground black pepper

1 pinch Italian seasoning

2 Tbsp all-purpose flour

1 Tbsp olive oil

1 c mushrooms, sliced

1/2 c dry Marsala wine

1/2 c fat-free, reduced-sodium chicken broth

2 Tbsp fresh-squeezed lemon juice

1 Tbsp fresh parsley

*Preparation:*

1. Gently pound chicken breasts to 1-inch thickness using a meat mallet.
2. Sprinkle both sides of chicken with salt, pepper, and Italian seasoning.
3. Place flour in a shallow dish. Dredge chicken in flour, coating both sides.
4. Heat olive oil in a large nonstick skillet over medium-high heat. Brown chicken breasts for about 3 minutes and remove from skillet.
5. To the skillet, add mushrooms, wine, chicken broth, and lemon juice. Reduce heat. Allow the sauce to simmer for 10 minutes.
6. Add chicken to the skillet and cover. Cook for an additional 5 minutes or until chicken is done. Use a meat thermometer to ensure doneness; chicken should be 165°F.

7. Sprinkle with parsley and serve.

\* *Squeeze additional lemon juice over the chicken before serving, if desired*

### Steamed Broccoli with Garlic

*4 servings*

1 bunch broccoli

1/2 tsp minced garlic

*Preparation:*

1. Rinse broccoli and break into bite-sized florets. Remove stems and cut in half or quarters.
2. In a saucepan, bring about an inch of water to a boil. Add broccoli, cover, and let cook until broccoli turns a bright green.

*\*Dress broccoli in any seasoning, if desired*

# 700 Calorie Dinner Menu
## *Chicken Marsala*

*4 servings*

4 (7 oz) boneless, skinless chicken breasts

1/4 tsp salt

1/4 tsp freshly ground black pepper

1 pinch Italian seasoning

2 Tbsp all-purpose flour

1 Tbsp olive oil

1 c mushrooms, sliced

1/2 c dry Marsala wine

1/2 c fat-free, reduced-sodium chicken broth

2 Tbsp fresh-squeezed lemon juice

1 Tbsp fresh parsley

*Preparation:*
1. Gently pound chicken breasts to 1-inch thickness using a meat mallet.
2. Sprinkle both sides of chicken with salt, pepper, and Italian seasoning.
3. Place flour in a shallow dish. Dredge chicken in flour, coating both sides.
4. Heat olive oil in a large nonstick skillet over medium-high heat. Brown chicken breasts for about 4 minutes and remove from skillet.
5. To the skillet, add mushrooms, wine, chicken broth, and lemon juice. Reduce heat. Allow the sauce to simmer for 11 minutes.
6. Add chicken to the skillet and cover. Cook for an additional 5 minutes or until chicken is done. Use a meat thermometer to ensure doneness; chicken should be 165°F.

7.  Sprinkle with parsley and serve.

* *Squeeze additional lemon juice over the chicken before serving, if desired*

### Steamed Broccoli with Garlic

*4 servings*

1 bunch broccoli

1/2 tsp minced garlic

*Preparation:*

1.  Rinse broccoli and break into bite-sized florets. Remove stems and cut in half or quarters.
2.  In a saucepan, bring about an inch of water to a boil. Add broccoli, cover, and let cook until broccoli turns a bright green.

*Dress broccoli in any seasoning, if desired*

# 500 Calorie Dinner Menu

*4 servings*

Be sure to begin your stir-fry with the vegetables that take the longest to cook so they are cooked until crisp-tender.

### *Veggie Beef Stir-fry*

3/4 lb sirloin steak, lean, boneless

1/3 c orange juice

2 Tbsp balsamic vinegar

2 Tbsp low-sodium soy sauce

2 Tbsp cornstarch

Cooking spray

1 tsp sesame oil

1 c red, orange, or yellow bell pepper and/or onions, chopped

1 c zucchini, squash, carrots, and/or bok choy, chopped

1 c mushrooms, snow peas, string beans, and/or water chestnuts

*Preparation:*

1. Trim off any visible fat from sirloin and cut into 1/4-inch cubes.
2. In large zipper-top bag, add sirloin and half each of the orange juice, balsamic vinegar, and soy sauce. Allow to marinate in refrigerator for 30 minutes.
3. In a bowl mix cornstarch and the remaining orange juice, balsamic vinegar, and soy sauce and set aside.
4. Heat nonstick skillet over high heat and coat with cooking spray. Cook meat for about 5 minutes and remove from heat.
5. Add sesame oil to skillet and begin stir-frying selected vegetables.
6. Add meat and second portion of marinade, and stir-fry for an additional 3 minutes. Sauce should thicken slightly.

# 700 Calorie Dinner Menu
## *Veggie Beef Stir-fry*

### *4 servings*

1 lb lean, boneless sirloin steak

1/3 c orange juice

2 Tbsp balsamic vinegar

2 Tbsp low-sodium soy sauce

2 Tbsp cornstarch

Cooking spray

1 tsp sesame oil

1 c red, orange, or yellow bell pepper and/or onions, chopped

1 c zucchini, squash, carrots, and/or bok choy, chopped

1 c mushrooms, snow peas, string beans, and/or water chestnuts

*Preparation:*

1. Trim off any visible fat from sirloin and cut into 1/4-inch cubes.
2. In large zipper-top bag, add sirloin and half each of the orange juice, balsamic vinegar, and soy sauce. Allow to marinate in refrigerator for 30 minutes.
3. In a bowl mix cornstarch and the remaining orange juice, balsamic vinegar, and soy sauce and set aside.
4. Heat nonstick skillet to high and coat with cooking spray. Cook meat for about 5 minutes and then remove from heat.
5. Add sesame oil to skillet and begin stir-frying selected vegetables.
6. Add meat and second portion of marinade, and stir-fry for an additional 3 minutes. Sauce should thicken slightly.

# 500 Calorie Dinner Menu
## *Pork Tenderloins with Thyme, Rosemary, and Sage Rub*

*6 servings*

2 (3/4 lb) pork tenderloins

2 garlic cloves, sliced

1 Tbsp water

1 tsp extra virgin olive oil

1/4 tsp salt

1/2 tsp freshly ground pepper

1 Tbsp dried thyme

1 tsp rubbed sage

1 tsp rosemary

*Preparation:*
1. Preheat oven to 400°F.
2. Trim any visible fat from the pork tenderloins, and cut 1/2-inch slits into the top of the pork. Stuff slits with garlic slices.
3. In a small bowl, combine water, olive oil, salt, pepper, thyme, sage, and rosemary. Season pork with rub mixture.
4. Place tenderloins in foil packet and place on the center rack in the oven. Bake pork for 30 minutes. Use a meat thermometer to ensure doneness; pork should be 160°F.
5. Slice pork tenderloins into 3-ounce servings and serve.

## *Beet Salad with Orange Vinaigrette*

*4 servings*

4 c fresh baby greens

2-1/2 c beets, shredded

2 oranges, sliced

3/4 Tbsp extra virgin olive oil

1-1/2 c shallots, minced

1/4 c vinegar

1/4 tsp ground black pepper

1/4 c chives, minced

*Preparation:*
1. Wash and dry baby greens and lay out on plate. Arrange the beets and oranges on top of the greens.
2. Heat oil in nonstick skillet over medium-high heat. Add shallots and vinegar, and cook for about 1 minute. Drizzle over salad and serve.

# 700 Calorie Dinner Menu
## *Pork Tenderloins with Thyme, Rosemary, and Sage Rub*

*6 servings*

2 (1 lb) pork tenderloins

2 garlic cloves, sliced

1 Tbsp water

1 tsp extra virgin olive oil

1/4 tsp salt

1/2 tsp freshly ground pepper

1 Tbsp dried thyme

1 tsp rubbed sage

1 tsp rosemary

*Preparation:*
1.  Preheat oven to 400°F.
2.  Trim any visible fat from the pork tenderloins, and cut 1/2-inch slits into the top of the pork. Stuff slits with garlic slices.
3.  In a small bowl, combine water, olive oil, salt, pepper, thyme, sage, and rosemary. Season pork with rub mixture.
4.  Place tenderloins in foil packet and place on the center rack in the oven. Bake pork for 30 minutes. Use a meat thermometer to ensure doneness; pork should be 160°F.
5.  Slice pork tenderloins into 5-ounce servings and serve.

## *Beet Salad with Orange Vinaigrette*

*4 servings*

4 c fresh baby greens

3 c beets, shredded

2 oranges, sliced

1 Tbsp extra virgin olive oil

1-1/2 c shallots, minced

1/4 c of vinegar

1/4 tsp ground black pepper

1/4 c chives, minced

*Preparation:*
1. Wash and dry baby greens and lay out on plate. Arrange the beets and oranges on top of the greens.
2. Heat oil in nonstick skillet over medium-high heat. Add shallots and vinegar, and cook for about 1 minute. Drizzle over salad and serve.

For the fish recipes, you may freely substitute other varieties from the list under "Other fish and seafood."

*Recipes developed by:*
*Tania Rivera, MS, RD, LD/N*
*Registered and Licensed Dietitian*

# Vitamins

I take mine every day. Rely on your doctor's advice. Supplementary vitamins are purposely absent in Dr. Siegal's Cookie Diet cookies and shakes mixes in the interest of taste, but all Weekly Boxes of both products include a supply of multivitamin tablets.

# Fluids

Drink lots of fluids, but let's not add calories. Two quarts (8 glasses) a day is good. Avoid juices. Water and flavored or carbonated waters with a couple of calories are OK. Diet sodas are also allowed if your doctor agrees. Coffee and tea are allowed, but don't add whitener.

# Weight

Think about the weight of the food you'll be eating. It's a good idea to have a little, inexpensive food scale in your kitchen. I've referenced so many ounces of this or that. Why guess?

# Summing Up

First, I might as well respond to a point that I know at least someone will raise. It will be pointed out that I am inconsistent when it comes to the specifics of the diet. I will be told, for example, that I allow red meat that certainly has some fat, yet I disallow certain fish that has even less fat than red meat. My critic deserves an answer.

As to that particular point, since I know that you will certainly be eating meat and, therefore, necessarily some fat, by eating low-fat fish, the fat calories overall are somewhat diminished.

Throughout the book, I assert that I am a practical man. That is to say, because of my long experience, I advocate what works, what I have seen consistently work. The diet that I advocate works whether the details are consistent or not.

In a way, I can still claim to be consistent because I am consistently inconsistent. Ponder that one!

By now, it should be clear that this is far from a starvation diet. More likely, you're wondering, "How am I going to eat all that food?" It's a lot, but remember what your day has been like up until dinner: no real food except cookies until dinnertime. The hunger control that you experience from the cookie makes it possible to last until dinner. By dinnertime, you *should* be hungry. I hope you'll be hungry. You have a big dinner to put away.

Are you beginning to see why this diet has been so successful? It's all about controlling hunger. If you add to your own motivation this tested method of hunger control, you have the recipe for weight-loss success.

# Chapter 22

# Keeping It Off

I started this book making the point that any method of taking off weight, and particularly Dr. Siegal's Cookie Diet, involves a considerable change in lifestyle. I'm going to end the book in a similar fashion.

Losing weight necessarily involves reducing your calorie intake sufficiently and for a measured period of time. Losing weight and maintaining it each requires a change in lifestyle, but a different one.

When you did Dr. Siegal's 28-Day Calorie Burn Rate Self-Test (found in the Resources section of CookieDiet.com), you should have come away after that first four weeks with a very good idea of what you need—what your caloric maintenance level really was. I use the past tense because that value probably changed substantially as the weight came off. As I noted in Chapter 13, that value changes as you lose weight and the test should be repeated periodically. If you tested yourself again when you were closer to your goal weight, you should have a reasonable estimate, taking into account your usual activity patterns, of how many calories a day it takes for you not to regain that weight.

How are you going to assure yourself that you are going to eat that many calories? Is there some structured plan by which you can accomplish that? Yes. There is a way that has worked for thousands. I'm going to show you how and I'm going to label it Plan A. As you may have guessed, Plan A involves eating cookies.

There also a Plan B and it's my preferred approach to maintaining weight. It's a lot less structured and restrictive than Plan A, and better for one's overall health. But having more freedom is not necessarily what works for most people who, I have learned, need to be told what to do. Nevertheless, in the hope that you are one of those disciplined enough to handle the freedom that Plan B affords, I'm going to tell you about it.

Plan B doesn't involve eating my cookies. In fact, it doesn't force you to follow any prescribed eating plan. But it does involve lots of aerobic exercise. Why exercise? Because the principle behind the plan is that you increase your need for calories (that is, your Daily Caloric Maintenance Level) by burning off extra calories through physical activity. As a result of this increase is your caloric requirement, in order to compensate for you additional calorie expenditure, you must eat more just to maintain your weight.

I know, it sounds like that same tired advice you've been hearing for years. You've been told that exercise is the key to losing weight and then maintaining it. Well, that's only a half-truth. The true part is the maintaining part. The part that doesn't work for most of us is the losing part.

There are a number of reasons why I insist that exercise is not an effective way to take off weight. The number one reason is that in practice, I have seen that it doesn't work, or at least it works for only a small number of those that embark on that method. For some who are carrying around as little as an extra 30 pounds or as much as 100 extra, that first exercise session is usually enough to send one to the showers ahead of schedule.

Anther reason is that the numbers don't add up. Consider this. Let's say that, when you started Dr. Siegal's Cookie Diet, your doctor advised that you eat 1,000 calories a day. Let's say that you determined, by testing, that your Daily Caloric Maintenance Level was 2,200 calories. That means that while dieting, you were creating a 1,200 calorie deficit each day. Were you to compare dieting with the amount of exercise you would have had to do in order to create a 1,200 deficit, you would immediately see that it would have been a daunting task. How long would you have to exercise to burn 1,200 calories? Probably, well over two hours every day. And what kind of exercise? Aerobic exercise. Jogging for two or more solid hours, or something else that was equivalent. Can you picture yourself doing that? For how many days a week, you ask? Every day. Yes, every day.

Are you beginning to see why exercise for weight loss doesn't accomplish the mission? While on Dr. Siegal's Cookie Diet, with your hunger comfortably controlled, you can manage to eat 1,000 calories a day, every day until the task is accomplished. You can achieve that 1,200 calorie deficit (or more). Do you think you are apt to be as constant if the alternative was to do two hours of grueling exercise every day?

Having shot down exercise as a weight-losing method, I'm now going to award it first place in the weight-maintenance competition. Plan B is indeed exercise. And if you recall, Plan B's job is to raise your maintenance level of calories with exercise. By doing so, you may now eat more calories and still maintain. Since the exercise you will be doing is necessarily aerobic, it will have an added benefit to your cardio-vascular system. It is even known to lower you cholesterol level. Nothing but benefits, nary a downside. It turns out that Plan B is my preference.

Still, it's not easy to sell Plan B to those who have just lost weight. No one doubts the benefit, yet many find Plan A preferable. For one thing, you don't sweat as much.

# Plan A: Dr. Siegal's Cookie Diet for Maintenance

Since you already know all about Dr. Siegal's Cookie Diet for weight loss, there is only a simple modification needed for weight-maintenance. You've been eating a 500 calorie dinner or a 700 calorie one or whatever has been recommended to you. The only change you are going to make for weight maintenance is to increase the calories at dinner.

By now you should have a pretty good idea of your Daily Caloric Maintenance Level. Perhaps you've tested it again recently. You are now going to switch to a dinner that brings your total daily intake up to that level. You'll still be eating the cookies during the day for hunger, just as before. But now your dinner will be what I could refer to as a "normal" dinner.

Suppose your caloric maintenance level is 2,000. Your six cookies contribute about 500. What you will eat from dinner until bedtime will have to amount to 1,500 calories. Are you surprised? Dinners of that size may have been your problem to begin with, but here's the difference. Your food up until that dinner (six cookies) only amounts to 500 calories.

I think it will be fruitless for me to designate rules for that dinner. I'm satisfied if I can convince people to eat according to set rules for a set period of time. During that time, I have an ally, the enthusiasm generated by seeing constant weight loss. I'm not that successful in dictating a lifetime of an eating regime. Maintaining one's weight, which necessarily means that the scale doesn't change much, doesn't foster that same type of enthusiasm. Being comfortable with a diet, without hunger, does enable one to stay within the rules.

There will be enough calories in that dinner to take it out of the weight-loss diet category. It will take some experimentation with amounts until you find the right quantity of dinner that allows you to maintain.

# Plan B: Exercise

Again, I prefer this method, even though for the most part you'll be saying goodbye to my cookies. I say for the most part because you can (and many people do) still enjoy them as a hunger-controlling snack food. But you won't need them to help you adhere to a low-calorie diet because you won't need to follow one with Plan B.

Plan B accomplishes the same thing as Plan A except that you are not given a set of eating rules that you might soon abandon. I have certain hopes. I hope you will be sensible and pit your eating habits in competition with your exercise habits. I hope you will emphasize protein in your meals (meat, poultry, fish). I hope you will continue to supplement with vitamins and drink lots.

Since Plan B is essentially exercise, and eventually rather demanding exercise, be sure you have checked with your doctor first, give him an idea of what you plan to do, and get his approval. He may choose to examine you and do certain tests to be sure you are a good candidate for aerobic exercise.

One of those heart rate monitors that joggers often wear is always a good idea. You can find them in virtually every sporting goods store. Your doctor should be able to tell you how to get the maximum benefit from it.

To make Plan B work, you'll need to burn up enough calories every day. I don't know what that number is because it will depend upon how much you are eating and how much you are exercising. In my own practice, I recommend starting with 500 calories a day of exercise. That's not that easy and the number is inexact because we truly don't know how many calories specific exercise burns per minute or per hour. It's a trial-and-error process, but you'll soon get good at it. Let's try for 500 calories per day.

In practice, I've observed that 500 will do it for most people. It raises their caloric maintenance level by that amount. Of course, anyone can be self-destructive and eat well over an extra 500 calories a day, but my experience is otherwise. Remember this instruction is for people who have reached their goal weight. I've mentioned earlier that among my patients, those who don't achieve a goal weight have little or no chance of maintaining. By the same token, there may be a mental phenomenon that takes over when someone does achieve normalcy—one that energizes his motivation to remain thin and healthy.

Of course, there are a variety of other activities that can be substituted for walking or running. Sports such as tennis, racquet-ball, and swimming will work. Golf won't cut it unless you turn off the golf cart and push it for 18 holes. Bowling? No way. Picture an hour of continuous and very hard work and ask whether your planned activity will meet that requirement.

You could go the route of seeking the help of a professional. A knowledgeable trainer or coach could be valuable. Be careful. Selecting the right one can be hazardous. You don't want one who received training at a single three-hour seminar or a two-day orientation at the gym. There are good people out there, but finding them is not easy.

To burn 500 calories per day will take something like a full hour of very fast walking or slow jogging. Needless to say, you won't be able to start flat out with that amount, and even if you chose to try, I don't recommend it. Start with the most minimal amount and work up to the full hour gradually. I wouldn't try to achieve that degree of daily activity in less than a month's time. But once you're into it, don't ever stop. That's what's going to keep you trim and healthy.

Getting back to Plan A (Dr. Siegal's Cookie Diet for Mainte-nance), I must confess that it was never my idea. It evolved as a result of my patients literally demanding it. One by one as each reached his or her goal weight they were told to discontinue the cookies and the single meal and get right into exercise (essentially

Plan B). You should have heard the objections. Those that were very honest said that they knew themselves and that they would never get into that much exercise. I had no choice but to allow them to stay on the diet with cookies and I adapted it so that the weight loss would turn into maintenance.

So what about a hybrid, a combination of the two plans? Well, why not? Regulate your intake by controlling hunger during the day with my cookies, eat a dinner that is completely satisfying and to your liking, and increase your caloric maintenance level with supplementary exercise. This may be the best of both worlds.

So there you have it. For weight loss , a temporary lifestyle change with cookies for hunger control and a reasonable dinner that will get you to a proper weight. Follow-up for maintenance with a different and permanent lifestyle, Plan A or Plan B or a combination of the two. When you succeed, it won't be because of luck. I don't like to talk of luck. It's dedication, not luck, that will bring you success. Nonetheless, "Good luck."

# Section Five

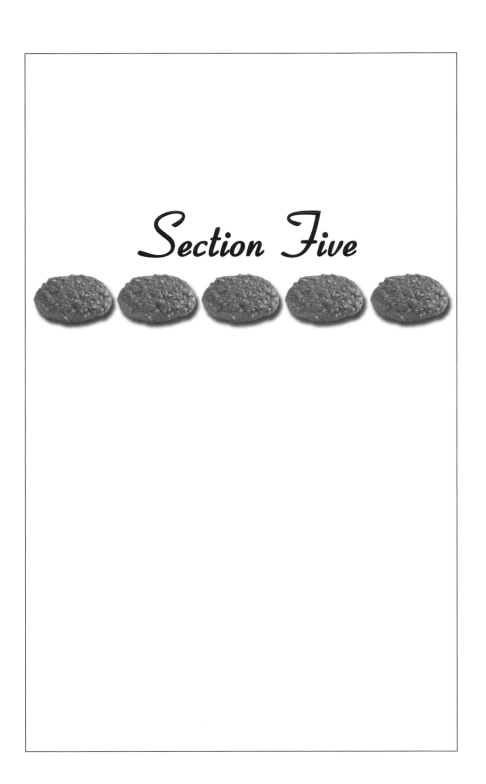

*Chapter 23*

# For Your
# Doctor's Eyes Only

This happens repeatedly. I'm told that Dr. Smith is on the line. I pick up.

"Dr. Smith calling from Podunk. I have a patient who wants me to monitor her on a weight-loss program. She brought in some cookies that have your name on the package. Can you tell me what this is all about?"

A proper response takes at least a good half hour.

This scenario happens frequently. Dr. Smith has a practice to run. He doesn't want my half-hour explanation; he wants a 60 second condensation. Since I also have a medical practice to get back to, I, too, can hardly afford the time. So I try to condense the explanation, but I can still tell—he's anxious to get back to his patients. I understand. Cookies? That would make any doctor skeptical.

I regularly invite physicians such as Dr. Smith to come and visit me and interact with me and my patients. I see a steady stream of these curious doctors. Of course, that's the best way to answer their questions, for them to view the whole process firsthand.

Doctor, what I'm not going to do is presume to tell you how to practice medicine or how to treat your patients. I will tell you what I do to help patients lose weight. You're free to take whatever you wish from my description, and perhaps you can even improve on it.

Here's a quick background. I've been treating overweight patients exclusively since before 1960. It's a big patient load—over the years more than half a million overweight patients. In the early days, I had a fair measure of success with my patients, but I also had my share of failures. I was not particularly satisfied with the percentages. By 1975 I had become increasingly troubled by the most common complaint of my unsuccessful patients: "I'm hungry." And this complaint often came from what appeared to be responsible, serious, motivated individuals. It was obvious to me that hunger wrecks diets. The appetite-suppressant medications that were available at that time helped, but they did not solve the problem. The medications that are available today are far less effective than those back then. Clearly, medications are not the answer.

In the seventies you might say that I became obsessed with constant complaints of hunger from my patients, and I turned my attention to investigating foods or, more properly, food components that seemed to influence hunger. It was obvious that all foods did not affect hunger the same. Clearly, some foods seemed to diminish hunger, while others seemed to stimulate it. Proteins seemed to fall into the former group, while carbohydrates belonged in the latter group. Fats also diminished hunger, but that seemed to have little value since fats contributed more than twice the calories of the other two food groups.

There was indeed a body of research relating to the subject of food substances and their relations to hunger. I was in the process of writing a book on the subject when it occurred to me to use what I had learned to engineer a food that was created specifically for satisfying hunger without supplying the abundance of calories contained in the popular snack foods. After a sizable effort, I came up with a formula, principally derived from combining and processing a group of food proteins to achieve a particular mix of amino acids. It didn't take long to settle on a cookie as the ideal vehicle for my formula. Cookies have a lot going for them. First of all, people like cookies. They are small and portable. They don't require refrigeration in the short term. Why not cookies?

My first subjects were, of course, my family and friends. My experimentation went on for some time, and I tried many variations in the formula. When I thought I really had something that worked, I tried it on a few patients. I had no qualms about doing this. I was dealing simply with a food. There were no drugs, nothing unusual or foreign to the human organism. It was just food, just cookies.

It was a success. Nothing in my medical practice theretofore had produced such a good result with hunger. Eating my cookies simply took the edge off of their hunger. And that's all Dr. Siegal's cookie did. There was no magic, no burning of fat, no nonsense common to those products in weight-loss commercials. It just satisfied hunger.

I have emphasized that addressing hunger head-on was essential to successfully getting my patients to lose weight. Equally important was keeping them motivated by showing them fast results.

Most of my patients appear to be motivated when I first see them. Some of them seem so convincing. Their rhetoric is easy to believe, at least at first. They may look quite anguished and relate how their weight has left them desperate. Their personal lives, their social lives, their business lives are in shambles because of their weight. "If I could just lose weight, everything would be fine." That sounds sincere enough until I hear that next obstructive word, "But."

"But I entertain clients at lunch every day. If I don't do this, my income will suffer."

"But my husband and I like to go out on weekends and we have a good meal and a few drinks. I can't give that up. I'll lose my happy home."

"But if I don't have a good breakfast, I can't go on with the day. You'll have to allow that."

In these situations, I have to exert restraint. I diplomatically suggest that perhaps these are excuses. The truly motivated patient does not introduce these stumbling blocks on our first encounter.

True motivation is common in people who are really desperate, those who will do anything if they could just get thin. Those are the ones I can best work with.

Nonetheless, no matter how motivated, how dedicated, how sincere this plump gal sitting across from me is, if I can't do something about her hunger, she is destined to fail. I've seen it repeatedly.

That's what Dr. Siegal's cookie is for. It satisfies hunger. That's it. Hunger is the target.

To indulge in a bit of whimsy, a quite effective way to control our hunger is to eat a big meal—a rack of barbecued ribs, a hefty serving of French fries, and a couple of beers? That'll control hunger. Obviously, that's not a practical way to control hunger while losing weight. Of course, one needs to minimize hunger, but with a minimum of calories. My cookie certainly has calories but not the excessive calories that my patients typically munch on to decrease their hunger. That's why Dr. Siegal's Cookie Diet works.

The following has come to be axiomatic with me.

*The faster my patient loses weight, the better.*

Perhaps, that's not what you expected to hear. Isn't all that good advice out there that comes from the self-styled experts directed toward eating a balanced diet, using the government's food pyramid, modifying one's behavior by learning to eat properly, and other assorted platitudes? I don't have to recite any more of those trite phrases? You know them. That's the kind of nonsense that's brought us where we are today: the highest percentage of obesity ever (65 percent). If we keep adhering to that kind of advice, we may indeed eventually hit 100 percent.

It's not that those instructions wouldn't work (although in many cases they wouldn't); it's that no one will follow them. So why do all these do-gooders waste their collective breath giving such useless advice?

I fancy myself as "practical." I do what works, not what I or someone else *thinks* will work. I accept the world as it is. The government, smugly through its food pyramid, tells you what to eat. Have you had three cups of milk, cheese, and milk-based desserts yet today? That's just one of the six food groups that you are directed to have every day. Have you had your three ounces of whole-grain bread today? No cheating now—it must be whole-grain bread, not white. What are your chances of having such specific amounts of each of the six groups tomorrow? How about for the rest of your life?

What I do in my practice is what has worked and what will continue to work. It recognizes who my patients are and not what I or some ivory tower researcher would like them to be. They are imperfect specimens of the human race, just as I am. There are limitations on what they are apt to do, and it would be folly for me to impose the kind of dietary advice that's universally aimed at us, the advice that virtually no one is willing to follow. People won't do it. And weight-loss failure begets more failure.

So why do I advocate fast weight loss? *Motivation.* There is no stronger motivating factor for a patient than to see consistent and continuing weight loss. That's what keeps people dedicated.

Perhaps you've experienced the look of joy on the face of a patient as she steps on the scale for her weekly visit. She sees a loss of three pounds or four pounds. Sometimes it may be only two. She's now lost a total of 10 or 20 or 50. That's a lot better than she did on her last diet. That satisfaction provides enough mental fuel to get her to adhere to the diet for another week. Yes, weight loss is its own motivator, and the faster, the better.

But how about the downside to rapid weight loss? We've all heard about it. Every time I appear on a TV show, there will always be some "expert" there who was brought in to disagree with me. Presumably the show believes this will add a measure of "fairness" to the piece. Recently, on some network morning show, some doctor who I doubt had treated many overweight patients first advised me to retire before I pass out any more stupid advice. He then went on to list all the horrible symptoms that befall us when we lose weight too fast. Never mind that neither he nor I have ever seen a patient with any of those symptoms from losing weight rapidly. I'm sure that none of the few patients he's treated displayed those symptoms, nor did any of the half million of my patients.

He was simply parroting the nonsense that when uttered enough times begins to sound like truth. Just look around you. Just look at the two out of three who are fatter than they should be. That's the result of "sensible" dietary advice. Who cares if that advice *would* work if it were followed. The point is that no one follows it, and therefore, it doesn't work.

Let's get back to the point of all this. I declare that fast weight loss monitored by a caring physician is perfectly safe. *Slow* weight loss, which generally is equivalent to *failed* weight loss, which results in *no* weight loss, is what's really dangerous. I'm not going to bore you with the statistics that you've already been hammered with. Obesity kills!

So what's a good way to accomplish fast weight loss? Total fasting is dangerous and does not even produce the fastest weight loss. We all know that the body has a very effective mechanism of slowing down the metabolism when we get no food at all. This minimizes the weight loss and keeps us alive somewhat longer. Of course, eventually we start metabolizing our own protein (our muscles), and that's not good.

What does work for fast weight loss and is really safe? The answer is a quite-low-calorie diet. Of course. That's obvious. But it doesn't work unless hunger is controlled.

What follows is not a set of instructions for you to follow in treating your patients. Again, I will not presume to teach you how to practice medicine. I'm simply going to tell you what I do in my practice, what I've done for perhaps more years than you have been in practice, what I've found works, and what I believe benefits patients immeasurably. What follows is not detailed. It's really a brief summary; I just want you to have a general idea. We all adapt our practice methods to our own particular biases.

First on the agenda for a new patient is lab work. I like to have that out of the way and have the results before I first see the patient. It's the kind of routine blood work you would expect. I do like to know if I have a diabetic on my hands, so I do a glucose tolerance, although I think that just a fasting glucose and a two-hour postprandial gives me the information I need. An EKG is a must. I also have the new patient fill out a general history form so I have a base line for my future questions.

The history and physical is rather routine. The history is helpful and gives me material to expand on in my questioning. Sometimes the H&P allows me to discover a lot of things for which I refer the patient to other physicians. Since I concentrate on the weight problem, I often end up cooperating with other physicians in getting the weight off.

The explanation of the diet and the rules that go along with it are extremely important. The instructions cannot be repeated too much. Our patients are told the nature of the diet when they first call and make an appointment. It's explained again by our staff on their first visit. We even play an audio tape to reinforce it. After examining the patient, I play a video of my giving them step-by-step instructions. And if that isn't enough, I personally go through the instructions again. Believe me; all this repetition isn't wasted. After all this effort, there is still a 50/50 chance they'll get it wrong. But that's OK. The advice will be repeated at each visit.

In my own practice, I routinely put patients on an 800 calorie diet. If you've had little experience with very low-calorie diets, you might be more comfortable with 1,000 calories or even 1,200 a day. They will lose quite well at the 1,000 calorie level. Later you may choose to become more aggressive.

At this point it's important to note that these patients are told to return each week for evaluation and, in fact, if they feel there is any problem, to call us immediately. Although these calls are rare, it gives them confidence to know that we choose to monitor them very closely, to check their progress or in some cases to delve deeply into their problems.

Our patients are given this instruction: *Eat the cookies when you're hungry.* That simple advice is all that the patient needs to remember. Of course, we may elaborate with something such as this: "The cookies are for satisfying hunger. That's their entire purpose, so eat them when you're hungry. When hunger strikes, eat a cookie. Wait about 15 minutes. If you can honestly say you're still hungry, eat a second. You should never need a third."

The patient is told that six cookies provide about 500 calories, and that is the number that is required every day: six cookies per day—no more, no less.

They are also instructed to eat or drink nothing else that has calories the entire day until dinnertime.

All their additional calories will come from dinner. Your own judgment should tell you what total calorie count for the day is appropriate. If their total calorie count for the day is to be 1,000, then the dinner will be 500. That can be a surprisingly ample dinner.

I'm purposely going to skip the details of the dinner so as not to be repetitious. You'll find a complete explanation in Chapter 21.

I know that those simple instructions will translate into faster weight loss than this patient has ever experienced. Along with this will come bolstered motivation and, for the first time, an actual expectation that the goal can be reached.

Of course there are some details that are passed on to the patient. Drink plenty of liquids. Water is preferable. Diet sodas are tolerated. Here's one that troubles a lot of our patients: coffee must be black and have no sugar. I allow artificial sweeteners, but you may have other ideas. However, they can have no milk or cream or anything else to lighten the coffee. I've yet to find any product in the supermarket to lighten coffee that has no carbohydrate (the enemy), so the coffee must be black. Patients complain a bit, but they generally accept that the sacrifice is worth it when they see the benefit.

The goal is to have no additional carbohydrate up until dinner. The smallest amount seems to work against the hunger-satisfying effect we're trying to achieve. Therefore, they should have no chewing gum or even supposedly sugar-free mints or other such products. These generally contain sorbitol, mannitol, or xylitol, which I have found to conflict with our objectives. In fact, they are admonished to eat and drink nothing but cookies and approved fluids until dinner. Nothing.

If all this sounds very rigid, then you obviously have gotten the message. Is this austere approach really consistent with motivating the patient? I've found that once you get to that first weighing one week after the patient starts the diet, the major hurdle is over. She can't wait to repeat that performance in the week that follows.

We repeat this same scenario, week after week as the pounds melt away. In most cases there will be lapses. They don't generally occur early in the treatment. But when self-satisfaction begins to set in, it becomes a dangerous time. Our overweight patient has now lost a considerable amount, yet she still has quite a bit to go. The desperation that she felt on the day she started the diet has now faded, and she is quite pleased with her improved shape. That's dangerous. Her overall outlook on life has changed so much that the motivation that got her to this point has waned. Here is where I must become extremely forceful and convincing.

My best weapon is to convince her of something that I know is absolutely true. After a few hundred thousand patients, I began to formulate rules that I now know are axiomatic. Here is one that I believe to be so true that I would bet the farm on it:

*My dear patient, you will never maintain your weight unless you first get to your proper weight.*

I can't begin to tell you how many times I have had a patient who has lost a tremendous amount of weight, perhaps 100 pounds or more, one who has become so self-satisfied that she elects to give up the struggle. She still has another 20 or 30 pounds to go, but that now seems unimportant to her. She is clearly a new woman, and she is reveling in it. What a shame! If she gives up the battle, I can bet that a year or so from then, I will see her again, probably 50 pounds or so heavier, and we'll start all over again. She'll have no problem with starting over because she knows it will work, but had she not given it up, her odds of maintaining would have been infinitely better. Maybe next time she'll make it to the goal.

Don't conclude that everyone who reaches the goal weight automatically maintains it. That is not at all what I'm proclaiming. What I'm saying is that a patient who reaches the goal weight has a fighting chance of maintaining it. The others don't seem to have the chance of a snowball in a very hot climate.

*My dear patient, you will never maintain your weight unless you first get to your proper weight.*

Don't ask me why my axiom is true. I don't know the reason. I don't know everything. I can come up with a lot of guesses, but I'm just reporting my observation. You're free to speculate just as I have.

As for weight maintenance, if you're really fascinated by all this, go to Chapter 22. This chapter is long enough.

# Index

For more information
about Dr. Siegal's Cookie Diet, visit

CookieDiet.com

or call

877-377-4342 (North America)
001 703-677-8068 (Elsewhere)

www.CookieDiet.com